guess
what came
to dinner?

guess
what came
to dinner?

PARASITES AND YOUR HEALTH

2nd edition

ann louise gittleman, m.s., cns

Avery
a member of
Penguin Group (USA) Inc.
New York

Appendix on pages 146–157 reprinted with permission from *The Medical Letter*.

Most Avery books are available at special quantity discounts for bulk purchase for sales promotions, premiums, fund-raising, and educational needs. Special books or book excerpts also can be created to fit specific needs. For details, write Penguin Group (USA) Inc. Special Markets, 375 Hudson Street, New York, NY 10014.

a member of
Penguin Group (USA) Inc.
375 Hudson Street
New York, NY 10014
www.penguin.com

Library of Congress Cataloging-in-Publication Data

Gittleman, Ann Louise.
Guess what came to dinner? : parasites and your health / Ann Louise
Gittleman.—Rev. and updated ed.
p.   cm.
Includes bibliographical references and index.
ISBN 1-58333-096-8
1. Parasitic diseases—Popular works.   I. Title.
RC119.G58   2001   00-069517
616.9'6—dc21

Printed in the United States of America

7   9   10   8

Book design by Meighan Cavanaugh

acknowledgments

I truly must thank my beloved mentors for their pioneering work in the arena of parasitology. My most sincere thanks to Dr. LuCrece Dowell, Dr. Hermann Bueno, Dr. Louis Parrish, Dr. Leo Litter, Dr. Peter Weina, Dr. Hazel Parcells, Dr. Robert Bradford, and Dr. Omar Amin. I am also grateful for the contibutions made by Reverend Hanna Kroeger, Dr. Fred Houston, Dr. Bernard Jensen, Ann Wigmore, Dr. Stuart Russell, Linda Hooper, and Herbert Shapiro. I especially want to thank the entire Schoor family, especially Michael, William, and Jo Len, for their total health vision. I would also be remiss if I did not thank Lyle Hurd and Roon Frost, who have always been huge supporters of my message.

Both Ann Castro and Stuart K. Gittleman provided invaluable assistance for this updated version of *Guess What Came to Dinner?* Alice Q. Swanson assisted me single-handedly with the original manuscript and I will forever be grateful for her diligence, compassion, and integrity. Alice is simply the best.

And of course I would like to acknowledge everyone at Penguin Putnam and Avery, especially Laura Shepherd and Christopher Mariadason, for their invaluable editorial assistance.

Most of all I would like to acknowledge you, my readers, whose letters, e-mails, and phone calls have made my research into the world of parasites a most fulfilling and worthwhile venture.

contents

foreword

As a professor of parasitology, founder of the Parasitology Center, and an international authority in the field with over 130 major publications and books on parasitology, I have not come across a book like Ann Louise Gittleman's *Guess What Came to Dinner?* It is the first published work that brought good science to the public in a user-friendly way. I was impressed upon my first reading of this book with how the subject of parasitic infections and diseases, not quite a dinner-table conversation topic, gracefully addressed both laymen's and practitioners' concerns.

Most significantly the book brought to the public's attention the importance of parasites and how they impact human health. If you think that, in the United States, we are safe from such third-world infections, then you are greatly misinformed. Some estimate that about 50 million American children are infected with worm parasites, only a small portion of which are detected and reported. This is particularly worrisome when one recognizes that microscopic, single-celled protozoans make up about 90 percent of all parasitic infections in the U.S. according to the Centers for Disease Control and Prevention (CDC). If existing parasitic infections are evenly distributed, there would be more than enough parasites for every living person to have one.

For one book, *Guess What Came to Dinner?*, to pioneer the effort to educate the public about such a problem is quite an accomplishment. Parasite infections can and do compromise our immune systems and digestive tracts, as well as all other organ systems. They can cause chronic fatigue, leaky gut syndrome, dysbiosis (imbalance of the intestinal bacteria), irritable bowel syndrome, fibromyalgia (sleep disorder), ulcerative colitis, allergies, toxicities, and many others. The point is, the situation is not improving.

Contributions like those of Ann Louise Gittleman are indispensable in order to manage this serious threat to our health. Her book includes sections on symptoms, types of parasites, how we contract parasitic infections, diagnosis, treatment, and prevention. I find the table of "Warning Signs" to be particularly useful and comprehensive. This second edition is especially valuable as it is updated and has incorporated many new and key research findings in practically all sections of the book. As a result, some changes and rearrangements were made that produced a very readable and informative version.

I must state that *Guess What Came to Dinner?* contributes considerably more to the public's understanding and awareness of the parasitic problem than many published hard-core scientific publications. It also provides a practical guide to how to deal with the problem both to the laymen and the practitioner.

Dr. Omar M. Amin, Ph.D.

preface

When I first wrote *Guess What Came to Dinner?* back in 1993, many people found the whole idea of parasites living inside a human host, well, quite shocking to say the least. Thankfully today, however, the general public has come to realize the cold, hard fact: Parasites are not only alive and well but thriving among (and in) a good sector of the American population. Parasites invade our homes, workplaces, day-care centers, restaurants, produce aisles, water resources, pets, and just about any other place we eat, sleep, or play. Some of them are pathogenic; all of them destroy our health and well-being. And the chilling truth is, parasitic infections are continually on the rise. Perhaps never before has it been more crucial for each of us to take action than right now.

Which is why I felt compelled to update this book. Recognizing the imminent need to empower people in the fight against parasitic infections, I've set out to enlighten readers with the latest findings. As I shared in the first edition, there are definite steps we must all take to eradicate the parasitic problem in our country. That hasn't changed. It begins with education and more definitive methods of detection, followed by specific, nutritionally supportive modes of treatment. And, of course, we also must gain savvy in our preventative process. This revision is designed to help you do all of that. You'll discover new information on various parasite species; breakthrough methods of detection, such as the stool antigen test; the most recent listing of antiparasitic drugs and treatment dosages from "The Medical Letter"; the latest herbal cures; as well as more helpful additions to the prevention tips.

Back when I wrote the original *Guess What Came to Dinner?*, a woman who typed the first draft of the manuscript remarked, "You ruined my life!" She then proceeded to relate to me that thirty-one years ago, her infant son had been infected with pinworms. The manuscript had brought back all the feelings she had buried . . . repulsion at first discovering these little thread-like worms wiggling in her son's diaper . . . not wanting to touch her own baby . . . feelings of somehow being a "bad" mother. But she didn't ignore the situation, nor was she in denial. She sought help not only for her baby, but for her whole family, and instituted a periodic deworming for all the children throughout their childhood.

It is my hope in writing this book that once you realize the extent of the parasite epidemic in America today, you will react as did my typist and take the proper measures, from diagnosis, to treatment, to prevention. I suggest you take this book to your doctor so that he can also be informed about this emerging health crisis.

The first part of the book will introduce you to the major reasons parasites are found in America today, what they are, how they do their damage, and how to recognize their symptoms and effects on the body. Then there will be discussions of the most common methods of transmission, from food and water to pets and day-care centers. The final chapters deal with ways to diagnose, treat, and prevent parasites. A special parasite-risk questionnaire is included for you and your doctor. A glossary is provided to help you become familiar with the jargon, and the appendix provides drug information for your doctor.

I hope that after reading this book, you will come away with a greater understanding of how we all are at risk for parasites, and what each individual can do to reduce that risk.

My own interest in parasites goes back to 1974 when one of my nutrition mentors, Dr. Hazel Parcells, first made me aware that parasites could be a very real, and very prevalent, problem in mainstream America. Since that time, I have clipped, collected, written away for, and acquired enough information on worms to fill several filing cabinets.

In 1984, I was interviewed on the subject of parasites by a national health magazine. The enormous response to that interview brought many concerned individuals to my office. I have since referred hundreds of people to doctors and laboratories for parasite testing, and my own practice has become overwhelmingly devoted to the nutritional implications of parasitic diseases.

Over the years, I have seen a multitude of patients with symptoms of chronic fatigue, hypoglycemia, food allergy, spastic colon, and respiratory disorders get well when parasites were eradicated from their systems. I feel that many individuals with unexplained health problems can benefit from a book of this kind.

Ann Louise Gittleman, M.S., CNS

introduction

Do you feel tired most of the time? Are you experiencing digestive problems—gas, bloating, constipation or diarrhea—that come and go but never really clear up? Do you suffer from food sensitivities and environmental intolerances? Have you developed allergic-like reactions and can't understand why? Are you depressed? Do you have difficulty gaining or losing weight no matter what you do? Have you even tried a yeast control program that helped to some degree but know you can't stay away from bread, alcohol, fruit, and fruit juices all your life? Do you sense something is not quite right with you but just can't figure out the cause—and, for that matter, neither can your doctor?

If these symptoms and feelings sound familiar, then you may be an unsuspecting victim of the parasite epidemic that is affecting millions of Americans. It is an epidemic that knows no territorial, economic, or sexual boundaries. It is a silent epidemic of which most doctors in this country are not even aware. Yet, according to parasite expert and medical researcher Louis Parrish, M.D., at least eight out of ten of his patients have some kind of parasite infection.

Here is the untold story that finally solves the mystery of many chronic health disorders. It is a story that began for me back in 1974 when I stumbled upon the connection between parasites and disease. In that year, at a special class for the study of "scientific nutrition" in Albuquerque, New Mexico, instructor Hazel Parcells, D.C., N.D., Ph.D., introduced the topic of worms in a most visual manner. She showed the class various preserved specimens of internal visitors that had been passed by patients undergoing treatment for a wide array of unresolved health problems. I have never forgotten the sight of those little bottles and what was in them. For the next two years, I refused to eat in any restaurants—for reasons you will read about later in this book. But most important, what I learned from Dr. Parcells was that worms, from the microscopic amoeba to the feet-long tapeworm, are a fundamental root cause of disease and are associated with health problems that go far beyond gastrointestinal-tract disturbances.

Since then, in my own nutritional practice, I have observed that many unexplained health conditions often disappeared when parasites were eliminated from the body. These conditions included environmental illness, skin problems, digestive problems, excessive fatigue, hypoglycemia, arthritic-like aches and pains, long-standing obesity, and even depression. Painstaking examination of my clients' food habits, favorite ethnic restaurants, lifestyle, and travel records often revealed the source of infection. I was amazed to find that a patient's travel history was often the missing key to unlocking the underlying cause of persistent flu-like symptoms, allergy, fatigue, gas, and intermittent constipation and diarrhea. Frequently, symptoms started shortly after a vacation to tropical islands, Asia, or South America or a camping trip in Colorado.

A central problem in solving the parasite puzzle is that many parasite-based illnesses can mimic diseases more familiar to the doctor. Roundworm infection, for example, has been misdiagnosed as peptic ulcer, and amoebic colitis is often mislabeled as ulcerative colitis. Chronic fatigue syndrome and yeast infection may really be a case of chronic giardiasis, while diabetes and hypoglycemia can be caused by tapeworm infection. The majority of doctors in the United States do not recognize parasites and therefore do not diagnose them. This may be due to the fact that parasitology courses in medical schools are usually offered by a tropical diseases department, giving rise to the notion that parasites are primarily a foreign concern. Furthermore, the inability of technicians to accurately diagnose the problem compounds the issue. The parasites' own reproductive cycle, in which eggs or cysts are passed at irregular intervals, also makes accurate diagnosis tricky.

Today, parasites and the diseases they cause are no longer found just in faraway places like the tropics—places that conjure up images of poverty and poor hygiene. Some parasites, like giardia and pinworms, are, in fact, found predominantly in temperate climates. These organisms as well as others have become more prevalent in America because of a number of modern-day factors discussed throughout this book.

The idea of harboring a living organism inside our bodies is repulsive and unpleasant to dwell upon, but learning all we can about our unwelcome boarders is the only way we can discover enough to evict them and rid ourselves once and for all of their presence. This is one situation in which ignorance is definitely not bliss.

knowledge is the key

In this book I will tell you:

- which twentieth-century factors have increased the parasite risk in the United States.
- what parasites look like and what symptoms to look for.
- how parasites are transmitted through food, water, animals, sexual practices, and day-care centers.
- how parasitic infections should be diagnosed.

In the following chapters, you will find answers to such questions as:

- What are the most effective natural and medical treatments for parasitic infection?
- How can my family and I prevent infection and reinfection?
- What lifestyle and travel precautions should I take?

The answers to these questions and many more may surprise and even shock you. But this book was written to do just that—awaken you, your family, and your doctor to the fact that parasites are alive and well and thriving in America today. I wrote this book because as a health-care professional I am worried . . . worried that so many individuals are not well, even though they are following a balanced diet and a good exercise program, and are unable to find the reason. I am convinced, after dealing with patients for more than eighteen years, that one of the major reasons for the chronic ill health we are seeing today is none other than parasites.

After you read this book, I urge you to share it with as many people as you can. Pass it on to your neighborhood health clinic, the hospital emergency room, your personal physician, and to veterinarians, day-care centers, outdoor clubs, restaurant owners, and travel agents. Education is the most potent weapon against the parasite epidemic. It is my hope that *Guess What Came to Dinner?* will become a wake-up call for every individual living in America today.

1

what you don't
know *can* hurt you

April 1999: A tiny parasitic worm that bores into tadpoles and
disturbs cells may be the cause of a large numbers of mysterious frog-leg deformities.

September 1998: The parasite *Cryptosporidium* causes widespread water contamination in Sidney, Australia.

May 1997: Business executives in Houston, Texas, fall prey to
the parasite cyclospora after eating infected produce.

April 1997: Centers for Disease Control estimates between
100,000 and 1,000,000 cases of *Giardia lamblia* occur each
year.

October 1994: NBC television program *Dateline* reports that
unnecessary deaths and illnesses throughout New York City
are the fault of cryptosporidium-contaminated water.

November 1993: According to a National Institute of Allergy
and Infectious Disease (NIAID) press release, parasites in
the U.S. affect millions.

Spring 1993: As reported by the NIAID, 100 deaths and more
than 400,000 residents become seriously ill in Milwaukee,
Wisconsin, after the parasite cryptosporidium contaminated
the water supply.

guess what came to dinner?

January 1993: Several deaths and hundreds of others fall ill to an
  E. coli outbreak in Washington due to fast-food hamburgers.

September 1992: Pork tapeworm cysts show up on the brains of
  four orthodox Jews: A feature story by the Associated Press
  zeroes in on the mystery.

Spring 1991: U.S. suspects Gulf War GIs are carrying the parasitic disease leishmaniasis and stops them from donating
  blood!

Believe it or not, Americans today are host to more than 130 different
kinds of parasites, ranging from microscopic organisms to foot-long
tapeworms. Practically every imaginable kind of exotic parasitic disease has
been found on our shores: African sleeping sickness, toxoplasmosis, schistosomiasis, giardiasis, amebiasis, filariasis—unpronounceable to most of
us, but potentially deadly nevertheless. Even malaria is making a come-
back, with cases of this mosquito-borne tropical disease being reported as
close to home as New Jersey, Virginia, Texas, and California.[1]

Parasites are an insidious public health threat in the United States today. Insidious because so very few people are talking about parasites, and
even fewer people are listening. Insidious because of the common misconception, among physicians and the general public alike, that parasites occur
only in tropical Third World countries, areas traditionally associated with
malnutrition and poor hygienic practices. Insidious because physicians do
not suspect, and therefore do not recognize, classic symptoms. And insidious because even if physicians are aware of the threat, most use outdated
and inadequate testing procedures, which result in underdiagnosis.

Lack of education is to blame. In the United States, physicians are simply not educated in parasitology and are, therefore, inexperienced in recognizing common clinical symptoms. A doctor's introduction to parasitology
may come from a chapter here and there in a microbiology course in medical school. If parasitology itself is taught at all, it is as a specialty in the department of tropical medicine at some universities. Courses in these
departments are not often elected by medical students who believe they
will not be seeing "tropical medicine" problems in their general practices in
the United States.

Yet, times have changed and parasites are much more widespread than previously believed. An article appearing in the June 27, 1978, *Miami Herald* states that a nationwide survey conducted by the Centers for Disease Control (CDC) in 1976 revealed that one in every six people selected at random had one or more parasites. The survey also pinpointed a parasite known as *Giardia lamblia* as the number-one culprit in water-borne disease. Louis Parrish, M.D., a New York City physician who specializes in parasites, wrote in 1991, "Based upon my experience, I estimate in the New York metropolitan area that 25 percent of the population is infected. . . ."[2] Projections for the year 2025 suggest that more than half of the 8.3 billion people on Earth will then be infected with parasitic diseases.[3]

Often regarded as opportunistic invaders, parasites have no respect for class boundaries. The publicized illnesses of celebrities like actor Yul Brynner, who became seriously ill from trichinosis after eating in a well-known New York restaurant, and tennis pro Martina Navratilova, who was affected by cat-transmitted toxoplasmosis, illustrate that we are all susceptible. Contaminated well water at some of this nation's most prestigious ski resorts has led to outbreaks of giardiasis, which goes to show that parasites can occur even in the seats of the mighty.

how did it happen?

A number of seemingly unrelated factors unique to the late twentieth century have contributed to the unrestrained parasite epidemic and added to the increased risk of parasitic infection. Some of these factors include:

- the rise in international travel.
- the contamination of municipal and rural water supplies.
- the increasing use of day-care centers.
- the influx of refugee and immigrant populations from endemic areas.
- the return of armed forces from overseas.
- the continued popularity of household pets.
- the increasing popularity of exotic regional foods.
- the use of antibiotics and immunosuppressive drugs.

- the sexual revolution.
- the spread of AIDS.

Let's examine each of these factors in detail.

INTERNATIONAL TRAVEL

Today more than ever before, American tourists are traveling to remote areas of the world. An affluent society is a mobile one. In 1990 alone, more than 390 million people worldwide made international trips for pleasure and/or business. Over 15 million of them were Americans, and half of these Americans traveled to Third World countries. More adventurous trips to exotic destinations like the Caribbean Islands and remote areas of Mexico, South America, Asia, Africa, China, and Israel have replaced the old-fashioned grand tour. We know that smallpox, cholera, and the plague have been eradicated, so we're safe.

Not so.

Unfortunately, travel can be fatal. As mentioned earlier, malaria, the most virulent of the parasitic diseases, is on the rise both here and abroad. Malaria is a ruthless killer, responsible for up to 2 million deaths per year in over 100 countries. The rise of this disease is partly due to the fact that mosquitoes have become resistant to DDT and other insecticides. And drug-resistant parasites have been found throughout South America, East Africa, and Southeast Asia. In parts of Thailand, the organism is resistant to every known drug, and the problem now presents a medical crisis.[4] There are many documented clinical cases of travelers, including businessmen and foreign exchange students, who had been infected in other countries but did not manifest symptoms until after their return home. In some of these cases, the disease was properly identified but by that time had progressed beyond the point of medical intervention, and the patients died.[5]

For the majority of us, less threatening conditions such as bouts of diarrhea are expected souvenirs of world travel. We pack out Pepto-Bismol right along with our passports and think nothing of it. Unless we go to St. Petersburg, Russia. Formerly known as Leningrad, this is "Giardia City" to visitors who go home with severe diarrhea, fevers, chills, muscle pain, and intestinal bloating. The cause: The city's tap water is infected with *Giardia lamblia,* a microscopic parasite. Visitors to Nepal are routinely stricken with severe cases of giardia, unaffectionately referred to as "Deli-Belly." Giardiasis, however, can do more than ruin your vacation. Symptoms of this illness can persist long after the vacation has ended. And it has been known to set the stage for unexplained conditions such as irritable bowel syndrome and chronic fatigue.[6,7]

Besides returning with photographs of the Great Wall of China, travelers there return with internal hitchhikers in the form of roundworms caused by widespread agricultural use of night soil (human waste). Eggs are not found in stool samples until sixty to seventy-five days after initial infection. By this time, they have gone through their pulmonary phase, creating such symptoms as cough, wheezing, bronchial spasms, and increased mucus. Symptoms of the intestinal phase may mimic those of peptic ulcer but require an entirely different treatment regimen.

The International Travelers Hotline of the Atlanta-based CDC warns those traveling to Africa of the danger of bathing, wading, or swimming in fresh water that may be infested with blood flukes, which cause a disease called schistosomiasis. This infection not only produces fever and chills, it elevates the number of specialized white blood cells known as eosinophils and causes abdominal pain with enlargement of the liver and spleen. Often, these symptoms do not show up until four to eight weeks after exposure, at which time the symptoms may be attributed to more familiar diseases with similar symptoms.

WATER CONTAMINATION

One of the greatest parasitic hazards is contaminated water—not only abroad, but right here in this country. A highly infectious parasite, *Cryptosporidium parvum,* is increasingly being recognized as the number one cause "in waterborne outbreaks in the U.S.A. and in children in tropical, developing areas . . . and [that] resists chlorine treatment and is easily spread in hospitals, daycare centers, and in impoverished households," according to a 1995 article in *Parasitology Today.*[8]

In 1993, malfunctions in the water systems of Milwaukee, among several other cities across the U.S., led to water-boiling advisories or shut-downs.[9] Apparently the invisible water-borne parasite cryptosporidium invaded the city's water supply, resulting in the illness of 400,000 people and the deaths of more than 100. According to a report that same year, one in four drinking water supplies tested in fourteen states was found to be contaminated with cryptosporidium.

The second most prevalent water-borne parasitic infection in the U.S. today is the *Giardia lamblia* parasite. David Addiss, M.D., a medical epidemiologist at the CDC, noted that giardiasis was mostly seen fifteen to twenty years ago in international travelers who drank from contaminated water supplies or in campers and backpackers who sipped from "pristine mountain streams" contaminated by infected forest animals or raw sewage. But that's all changed. Giardia—that traveling companion from Nepal and St. Petersburg—first surfaced here in the West and then spread to the Northeast, Southeast, Rocky Mountains, and California Sierras. Steven Rochlitz, Ph.D., states in his book *Allergies and Candida* that "Giardiasis may be a rampant problem in the U.S. today since 50% of our water supply is contaminated with it and, unlike bacteria, it is not killed by chlorination."

We must also factor in that hundreds of small water systems throughout the country do not have adequate purification systems. And in urban as well as rural areas, streams and watersheds can become contaminated through infected human sewage. Understandably, people are opting for bottled water and water filters to avoid parasitic infection.

However, the fact remains that parasitic infection via contaminated water may be much more prevalent than we think. A release from the National Institute of Health says "many parasitic diseases such as giardiasis and cryptosporidiosis are not always reported to health authorities, so that we suspect the extent and impact of parasitic diseases in the United States is underestimated."[10]

DAY-CARE CENTERS

Rampant parasitic infections exist in day-care centers nationwide. A 1997 *Wall Street Journal* article quoted one New York City pediatrician who was experiencing a definite increase in giardia outbreaks and "attributing the cases to exotic vacations and the growth of daycare for diaper-aged children."[11] When a child becomes infected in any of the ways discussed in this book, he can easily infect others in day-care centers. The Centers for Disease Control has estimated (estimated because exact figures are not known) that every year, day-care centers are the source of nearly 20,000 cases of giardiasis. A recent CDC survey found that in Fulton County, Georgia, approximately 25 percent of all children in day care were infected with giardia; in New Haven, Connecticut, the rate was twice as high at 50 percent; and in Anaheim, California, the rate of giardia in one day-care center increased from 3 percent to 43 percent from 1981 to 1991.[12]

Since the disease can be spread through direct contact with infected feces, day-care centers provide a ready environment for transmission and have been referred to as "the open sewers of the 20th Century."[13] Because giardia cysts lodge under the fingernails, the infection can be inadvertently spread from one infant to another during diaper changes. It is also spread by inquisitive toddlers touching dirty diapers and then contaminating toys, drinking faucets, and themselves with their frequent hand-to-mouth contact. According to Dennis Juranek, D.V.M., chief of Epidemiology and of The Parasitic Disease Branch at the CDC, roughly 20 percent of parents become infected themselves while caring for their sick children.

IMMIGRANTS

Parasitic infection is more predominant in the tropics and the subtropical areas of the world because of climate and unsanitary conditions. Parasites are much more prevalent in immigrants from areas like the South Pacific, Mexico, South America, Asia, and Haiti. Not counting illegal aliens, over 16 million foreign students, diplomats, travelers, and immigrants entered the United States in 1989. During the 1970s, at the end of the Vietnam War, this country was inundated with a massive influx of immigrants from Southeast Asia. Many of these refugees and immigrants came from parasite-infested areas. While they may not be exhibiting symptoms of the diseases, they may still be carriers, just as infectious as those with full-blown symptoms.

Recent immigrants to this country, who often are unskilled and unable to speak English but willing to work for minimum wages or less, very often seek jobs in kitchens where today there are no obstacles to their employment. I have observed that the majority of restaurant workers no longer wear hair nets or gloves when handling food, and often the same person who serves your food takes your "dirty" money. With this lack of basic sanitation in the restaurants of America, the exposure rate to infectious diseases is mushrooming.

Immigrants also find work as babysitters or housekeepers. An Associated Press article that ran on September 3, 1992, carries the headline "Worldly Worms! Traveling Parasites Leave Latin America to Afflict Big Apple." The article goes on to describe how four orthodox Jews in New York City were mysteriously stricken with seizures. CT scans showed pork tapeworm cysts in the brain, a most startling revelation considering these individuals never ate pork due to their religious dietary laws. A Centers for Disease Control formal investigation discovered the single common denominator in every case history—a housekeeper originally from Central America, where pork tapeworm infection is relatively common. The investigators theorized that the housekeepers unknowingly carried the tapeworm eggs and infected the Jewish families by contaminating their food.

ARMED FORCES

Soldiers stationed overseas can harbor a variety of parasites. More than the troops come home. Headlines such as "Disease Is Cited in Veterans Suit"[14] and "Gulf War Parasite Halts Troop Blood Drive"[15] graphically bring the awareness of parasitic diseases from foreign shores to America. From 1963 to 1975, thousands of troops returning from Southeast Asia were carrying parasite-induced diseases that affected their intestines, lungs, liver, and central nervous systems.[16] In 1985, five Vietnam War veterans filed a class-action medical malpractice suit against the Veterans Administration for failing to properly test, diagnose, and treat them for parasitic filariasis. Filariasis, a disease endemic to southeast Asia, is caused by worms carried by infected mosquitoes and can lead to swelling of the lymph glands and a condition known as elephantiasis. Lawyers and doctors for the five veterans contend that hundreds to tens of thousands of Vietnam veterans may be suffering from this disease. More recently, 540,000 American troops returning from Desert Storm were told not to donate blood because of the incidence of the parasitic disease leishmaniasis, spread by desert sand flies. Diarrhea, abdominal pain, and fever are symptoms of this infectious disease. Unexplained illness with fever may be a sign of a new species of leishmaniasis found in the Gulf vets.

PETS

Pets are hosts to numerous parasites and are unexpected spreaders of disease. There are 240 infectious diseases transmitted by animals to humans. Of these, 65 are transmitted by dogs and 39 by cats. There are 110 million dogs and cats living in America's households, making exposure to some of these diseases significant. Dogs, for instance, are known carriers of *Giardia lamblia,* which is easily picked up through ground water or from contact with animal waste. A regularly dewormed cat or dog can still pose a threat since the infections may recur. One pet-food manufacturer says that 89 percent of all house cats in America sleep with their owners. Dog and cat roundworm, hookworm, and cat-transmitted toxoplasmosis can become severe in pregnant women and children and even life threatening in immuno-compromised individuals. Phillip Goscienski, M.D., head of the Infectious Disease Branch of Pediatrics at the Naval Regional Medical Center, finds it remarkable that these diseases are almost always unsuspected and unrecognized.[17]

But dogs and cats aren't the only problem. A 1998 article in the *San Luis Obispo Telegram-Tribune* reported a one-year-old child was "hospitalized after being infected by a rare potentially deadly parasitic disease carried by raccoons . . . the child . . . apparently contracted the illness by ingesting microscopic roundworm eggs that are commonly found in raccoon feces."[18] The article also stated that the parasite can be transmitted by birds, rodents, and rabbits as well.

PROCESSED AND SUGAR-LADEN FOODS

Most of us in the U.S. love sweets. In fact, the average American consumes approximately 150 pounds of sugar each year. Yet, high-sugar diets are linked not only to type II diabetes, obesity, yeast infections, attention deficit disorder, and asthma but also implicated in the growing problem of parasites. Parasites thrive in a sugar-laden environment, which is why sugar in all its forms should be avoided. That means avoiding simple carbohydrates and eating a limited amount of complex carbohydrates, which elevate blood sugar and insulin levels.

Of all the macronutrients, both simple and complex carbohydrates create the cleanest burning fuel for energy. Sucrose and white sugar are simple carbohydrates, which are digested and absorbed fast and give a quick energy boost. Complex carbohydrates, on the other hand, consist of chains of simple sugars and are derived from starches, like grains, legumes, and starchy vegetables (squash and potatoes). Many complex carbohydrates take longer than simple sugars to digest and absorb. Consequently they enter the bloodstream more slowly than the simple carbohydrates, producing longer-lasting steadier energy.

A good rule of thumb is to follow the glycemic index, which rates carbohydrates by how rapidly they break down as sugar (glucose) in the bloodstream. Also, avoid the ever-popular low-fat, high-carbohydrate diets. They are excessively high in certain complex carbohydrates and low in high-quality protein as well as healthy fats. As a result, these diets directly contribute to the rise of parasitic infestation. And keep in mind that certain complex carbohydrates like corn, potatoes, brown rice, and whole wheat are absorbed quickly by our bodies in much the same way as simple sugars.

EXOTIC FOODS

The more cosmopolitan the city, the greater the proliferation of exotic restaurants. Our fascination with regional foods has led to an increased incidence of parasites. Exotic foods that are often prepared raw or undercooked pose a significant parasite risk. Sushi . . . sashimi . . . steak tartare . . . ceviche . . . Dutch herring. The CDC 1976 nationwide survey into parasitic diseases pinpointed a 100-percent increase in tapeworm infections in the preceding ten years. Tapeworm is transmitted in raw or undercooked fish, beef, and pork.

Pacific rockfish (commonly known as red snapper) and Pacific salmon are most frequently infested with anisakid worms, although the worms have also been found in Atlantic waters in other fish, such as haddock.[19, 20] With the increasing prevalence of microwave cooking, fish is frequently undercooked, allowing the larvae to survive and enter the human system. These worms cause anisakiasis (a condition resembling Crohn's disease), stomach ulcers, and appendicitis. Surgical treatment may be necessary in the later course of this disease because of intestinal perforation or obstruction.

In 1996 nearly 1,000 became ill due to an outbreak of the cyclospora parasite, which was traced to raspberries imported from Guatemala. Tainted raspberries from Guatemala and Chile also caused a wedding party to fall prey to the parasite cyclospora in 1997. And in 1998, dozens of Texas business executives became ill after a luncheon where at least six of them were infected with the cyclospora parasite.[21]

ANTIBIOTICS AND IMMUNOSUPPRESSIVE DRUGS

As mentioned before, parasites are opportunistic invaders. When the intestinal system is in healthy balance, there is less opportunity for parasitic infestation. Antibiotics, however, kill bacteria indiscriminately, both the good and the bad, upsetting the natural ecology of the gastrointestinal tract and vagina. This often leads to yeast overgrowth and trichomoniasis. *Trichomonas vaginalis* is a microscopic parasite that causes foul-smelling vaginal discharge, burning sensation, and inflammation. In some areas of the United States, this condition is found in 50 percent of all women. It is sexually transmitted and when passed to a male partner can cause non-specific urethritis.

The immune system is our first line of defense against invading bacteria, viruses, and parasites. Patients with compromised immune systems or those undergoing immunosuppressive drug therapies for cancer and organ transplants are at greater risk for toxoplasmosis, an opportunistic infection that attacks the central nervous system, heart, and lungs. While the effects of this infection in healthy individuals can be asymptomatic, in compromised patients it can be life threatening.

THE SEXUAL REVOLUTION

The sexual revolution of the late 1960s and early 1970s made it acceptable to have a variety of sexual partners and practices. The increase in the number of sexual partners also increased the likelihood of sexually transmitted parasites, which include *Trichomonas vaginalis, Entamoeba histolyticia, Giardia lamblia*, pinworms, and pork tapeworms. The increasing acceptance of anal/oral sex among heterosexuals has opened the door to the spread of parasite infections because many of these infections are spread to hands, mouth, and body via fecal contamination.

SPREAD OF AIDS

There seems to be a relationship between parasites and AIDS. Parasites may be a cofactor in the development of AIDS. An article appearing in the *New England Journal of Medicine* draws a connection between the disease and epidemic outbreaks of amebiasis two years prior to the San Francisco AIDS outbreak.[22] University of Virginia School of Medicine researchers point out that amoebas produce a substance that ruptures immune defense cells that have engulfed the HIV virus. Once those cells are ruptured, the virus spreads throughout the system. In addition, as a result of the AIDS epidemic, the incidence of many unusual parasitic diseases, such as *Pneumocystis carinii* pneumonia, cryptosporidiosis, and strongyloidiasis has increased. These diseases can be fatal in the AIDS victim.

our global village

As jet travel has transformed our planet into a global village, so, too, have parasites developed wings. Our current lifestyle habits of traveling, eating out, camping in the wilderness, placing children in day-care centers, caring for pets, and using antibiotics increase the likelihood of exposure to parasitic disease here in America.

On January 29, 1985, the Public Broadcasting Service aired a *Nova* program entitled "Conquest of the Parasites." In this televised documentary, the diseases that parasites cause were referred to as the "great neglected diseases." They are "great" because they affect hundreds of millions of people, and they are neglected by the public, by physicians, and by the political and funding agencies of the world. Although hookworm disease affects about 900 million people worldwide, the world's agencies spend less than $1 million on hookworm research. That's less than a dime per stricken individual, a particularly disheartening figure when one realizes that 60,000 of those stricken will die. Given the enormity of the parasitic infection problem, it is clear that funding is poorly allocated.

To prevent *you* from "neglecting" the diseases, this book will help you understand the kinds of internal parasites most commonly found in Americans today, the typical signs and symptoms, means of transmission, diagnostic procedures, and methods of treatment and prevention.

$$\mathcal{2}$$

the warning signs
of parasites

More than half of all Americans will at some point in their lives become hosts to parasites, according to health experts. Since the effects of infection reach far beyond the gastrointestinal tract, it behooves all of us to be on the alert for the wide array of bodily symptoms that signal the presence of parasites. Signs and symptoms may come about during initial exposure, shortly after that exposure, or many months later. What many of us are attributing to old age, stress, or plain old poor health, may, in fact, be due to an uninvited guest.

The word "parasite" is from the Greek words *para* (meaning beside) and *sitos* (meaning food). Most medical dictionaries define a parasite as "an animal or plant that lives on or in another organism from which it obtains nutriment." A basic element in the parasite definition is that a parasite is "usually injuring" or "without contributing to survival." The relationship that is formed between the two organisms is defined as "parasitism." My concern in this book is endoparasites, which live inside the body, rather than ectoparasites, which live on the body like mites and ticks. The organism that serves as the home for the parasite is known as the "host." The transmitting agent that carries the infecting pathogen is called a "vector."

The human being becomes a host through one of four pathways. The first is infected food or water (sources of roundworm, amoeba, and giardia);

the second is via a vector, such as a mosquito (carrier of dog heartworm, filaria, and malaria), a flea (carrier of dog tapeworm), the common housefly (transmits amebic cysts), and the sand fly (carrier of leishmaniasis); the third is from sexual contact (infected partners can transmit trichomonas, giardia, and amoeba); and the fourth is through the nose and skin (pinworm eggs and *Toxoplasma gondii* can be inhaled from contaminated dust; hookworms, schistosomes, and strongyloides can penetrate exposed skin or bare feet). The airplane can be considered another parasitic pathway or vector in its own right because extensive foreign travel has exposed Americans to a whole gamut of exotic diseases never before encountered in their homeland.

The table on page 22—which identifies the parasite, size, site in host, portal of entry, source of infection, most common symptoms, laboratory diagnosis, therapeutic agents, and special remarks—will help you see that practically every part of the human body can be affected by parasites. Most invaders inhabit the gastrointestinal tract (mainly the small intestine, but also the colon), with the circulatory system (blood and lymph) following close behind. During the adolescent or larva stages of their migratory life cycle, many organisms can invade the lungs. And organs like the heart, liver, spleen, eyes, and brain are not immune from the damaging effects.

While many of our unexpected visitors may be invisible, their symptoms can be very apparent. In this situation, the old adage "out of sight, out of mind" definitely does not apply. The warning signs for parasites are also symptoms of other common illnesses. For this reason, parasitic infections are often misdiagnosed, and ensuing treatment does not result in the alleviation of symptoms or disease. When symptoms continue even after a course of treatment, parasite screening procedures should be initiated. The following are warning signs for parasites: constipation, diarrhea, gas and bloating, irritable bowel syndrome, joint and muscle aches and pains, anemia, allergy, skin conditions, granulomas, nervousness, sleep disturbances, teeth grinding, chronic fatigue, and immune dysfunction.

constipation

Some worms, because of their shape and large size, can physically obstruct certain organs. Heavy worm infections can block the common bile duct and the intestinal tract, making elimination infrequent and difficult.

diarrhea

Certain parasites, primarily protozoa, produce a prostaglandin (hormone-like substances found in various human tissues) that creates a sodium and chloride loss that leads to frequent watery stools. The diarrhea process in parasite infection is, therefore, a function of the parasite, not the body's attempt to rid itself of an infectious organism.

gas and bloating

Some parasites live in the upper small intestine, where the inflammation they produce causes both gas and bloating. This situation can be magnified when hard-to-digest foods such as beans and raw fruits and vegetables are eaten. Persistent abdominal distension is a frequent sign of hidden invaders. These gastrointestinal symptoms can persist intermittently for many months or years if the parasites are not eliminated from the body.

irritable bowel syndrome

Parasites can irritate, inflame, and coat the intestinal cell wall, leading to a variety of gastrointestinal symptoms and malabsorption of vital nutrients, particularly fatty substances. This malabsorption leads to bulky stools and steatorrhea (excess fat in feces).

joint and muscle aches and pains

Parasites are known to migrate and encyst (become enclosed in a sac) in joint fluids, and worms can encyst in muscles. Once this happens, pain becomes evident and is often assumed to be caused by arthritis. Joint and muscle pains and inflammation are also the result of tissue damage caused by some parasites or the body's ongoing immune response to their presence.

anemia

Some varieties of intestinal worms attach themselves to the mucosal lining of the intestines and then leach nutrients from the human host. If they are present in large enough numbers, they can create enough blood loss to cause a type of iron deficiency or pernicious anemia.

allergy

Parasites can irritate and sometimes perforate the intestinal lining, increasing bowel permeability to large undigested molecules. This can activate the body's immune response to produce increased levels of eosinophils, one type of the body's fighter cells. The eosinophils can inflame body tissue, resulting in an allergic reaction. Like allergies, parasites also trigger an increase in the production of immunoglobulin E (IgE).

skin conditions

Intestinal worms can cause hives, rashes, weeping eczema, and other allergic-type skin reactions. Cutaneous ulcers, swellings and sores, papular lesions, and itchy dermatitis can all result from protozoan invasion.

• Protozoan Infections in People •

The information in this table can assist you and your doctor in identifying and treating parasitic diseases. Note that "Site in Host" refers to the part of the body in which the parasite "resides" permanently. Parasites normally migrate to this point after entering the host through the "portal of entry." When parasites are present in a human host, they produce a wide variety of symptoms, which can be as general as fever, chills, or intestinal problems. Diagnosis can

	Common Name of Parasite or Disease	Length of Parasite	Site in Host	Portal of Entry
NEMATHELMINTHES	**ROUNDWORMS**			
Necator americanus	New World or tropical hookworm Uncinariasis	To 1.1 cm	Small intestine, attached	Skin, usually feet
Ancylostoma duodenale	Old world hookworm Ancylostomiasis	To 1.3 cm		
Ancylostoma braziliense	Creeping eruption, cutaneous larva migrans (hookworm larva)	To 0.3 mm (larva)	Intradermal	Skin
Ascaris lumbricoides	Large roundworm	To 35 cm	Small intestine	Mouth
Toxocara canis T. cati	Visceral larva migrans	0.3 mm (larva)	Liver, lung, brain, eye	Mouth
Enterobius vermicularis	Pinworm, seatworm, Oxyuris	To 1.3 cm	Large intestine, appendix	Mouth
Trichuris trichiura	Whipworm, threadworm	To 5.0 cm	Caecum, large intestine, ileum	Mouth

not, therefore, be based upon symptomatology. Accurate diagnosis and identi-
fication of the parasite can be made only if the proper laboratory tests are administered and reliably interpreted. Treatment may then include surgical
and/or nutritional measures as well as drugs (see the Appendix for specific
drug recommendations).

Source of Infection, Intermediate Host or Vector	Most Common Clinical Symptoms	Laboratory Diagnosis	Therapeutic Agent	Remarks
Infective filariform larvae in soil	Anemia, growth retardation, G.I. symptoms	Eggs in stool	Pyrantel pamoate Bephenium-hydroxynaph-thoate Tetrachlorethy-lene Thiabendazole	Prophylaxis by excreta dis-posal. Iron therapy im-portant in blood regener-ation
Dog and cat hook-worm larvae in soil	Serpiginous skin lesions, itch	History and physical ex-amination	Thiabendazole ointment, freezing, X ray	Infection of bathers, plumbers, "sandbox" babies
Eggs from soil or vegetables	Vague abdomi-nal distress	Eggs in stool	Piperazine Pyrantel pamoate	Worms migrate into bile, pan-creatic ducts and peritoneum. Intestinal obstruction
Eggs from soil	Pneumonitis, eosinophilia	Hemagglutina-tion, floccula-tion tests	Prednisone Diethylcarbama-zine Thiabendazole	Eosinophilia, anemia, hyp-erglobulinemia
Eggs in environ-ment; autoin-fection	Anal pruritis	Eggs in perianal region. Scotch tape swab	Pyrantel pamoate Piperazine Pyrvinium pamoate	Entire family frequently in-fected. Per-sonal hygiene important
Eggs from soil or vegetables	Abdominal dis-comfort, ane-mia, bloody stools	Eggs in stool	Mebendazole Hexylresorcinol enema	Worm lives many years. Fre-quently with hookworm and Ascaris

	Common Name of Parasite or Disease	Length of Parasite	Site in Host	Portal of Entry
NEMATHELMINTHES **ROUNDWORMS** (*cont.*)				
Trichinella spiralis	Trichinosis	To 0.4 cm	Adult: small intestine wall. Encysted larva: striated muscle	Mouth
Strongyloides stercoralis	Cochin China diarrhea	To 0.2 cm	In wall of small intestine	Skin
Wuchereria bancrofti	Filariasis	To 10 cm	Lymphatics	Skin
Brugia malayi	Filariasis	To 6 cm	Lymphatics	Skin
Acanthocheilonema perstans	Persistent filaria	To 8 cm	Body cavities	Skin
Mansonella ozzardi		To 8 cm	Body cavities	Skin
Loa loa	Eyeworm	To 7 cm	Subcutaneous	Skin
Onchocerca volvulus	Blinding filariasis	To 50 cm	Subcutaneous	Skin
Dracunculus medinensis	Fiery serpent Guinea worm	To 120 cm	Subcutaneous	Mouth
PLATYHELMINTHES **TAPEWORMS**				
Taenia saginata	Beef tapeworm	To 12 meters	Small intestine	Mouth
Hymenolepis nana	Dwarf tapeworm	To 4 cm	Adults and cysts in small intestine	Mouth
Hymenolepis diminuta	Rat tapeworm	To 60 cm	Small intestine	Mouth

Source of Infection, Intermediate Host or Vector	Most Common Clinical Symptoms	Laboratory Diagnosis	Therapeutic Agents	Remarks
Infected pork, cyst (rarely bear)	Orbital edema, muscle pain, eosinophilia	Skin test, comp. fix., flocculation, biopsy	Prednisone gives symptomatic relief Thiabendazole	Thorough cooking of pork and pork products kills encysted larvae
Larva in soil	Abdominal discomfort, diarrhea	Larvae in stool	Thiabendazole Pyrvinium pamoate	Autoinfection occurs
Mosquitoes	Lymphangitis, fever	Blood smear, night	Diethylcarbamazine, surgery	Elephantiasis of leg, arms, scrotum, breasts
Mosquitoes	Lymphangitis, fever	Blood smear, night	Diethylcarbamazine, surgery	Elephantiasis
Culicoides (fly)	Abdominal pain due to liver invasion(?)	Blood smear	Diethylcarbamazine	
Culicoides (fly)	Asymptomatic(?)	Blood smear	Diethylcarbamazine	
Chrysops (fly)	Local inflammation, transient tumor	Blood smear, day	Diethylcarbamazine Surgical removal	Calabar swelling
Simulium (fly)	Subcutaneous nodules, loss of vision	Skin biopsy, nodule aspirate	Diethylcarbamazine Suramin	Nodules on head and body
Cyclops	Inflammation ulcers of legs legs and feet	Lesions, X ray of calcified worm	Thiabendazole Niridazole	Boil or filter drinking water
Cysts in beef	Usually none	Eggs and segments in stool. Scotch tape swab	Niclosamide Quinacrine Paromomycin	Usually only 1 worm
Eggs from feces	Abdominal discomfort	Eggs in stool	Niclosamide Paromomycin	Numerous worms, infection of children
Cycts from insects	Usually none	Eggs in stool	Niclosamide Paromomycin	Primarily a rat parasite

	Common Name of Parasite or Disease	Length of Parasite	Site in Host	Portal of Entry
PLATYHELMINTHES	**TAPEWORMS** (*cont.*)			
Diphyllobothrium latum	Fish or broad tapeworm	To 10 meters	Small intestine	Mouth
Taenia solium	Pork tapeworm	To 7 meters	Small intestine	Mouth
T. solium (cysts)	Cysticercosis Verminous epilepsy	To 0.8 cm; in brain, to 2.5 cm	Muscles, brain, eye	Mouth
Echinococcus granulosus	Hydatid cyst	To 15 cm	Liver, lungs, brain, bones	Mouth
PLATYHELMINTHES	**FLUKES**			
Schistosoma mansoni	Schistosomiasis "Bilharzia"	To 1.4 cm	Veins of large intestine	Skin
Schistosoma haematobium	"	2.0 cm	Veins of urinary bladder	Skin
Schistosoma japonicum	"	2.6 cm	Veins of small intestine	Skin
Fasciolopsis buski	Intestinal fluke	2–7cm	Small intestine	Mouth
Clonorchis sinensis	Human liver fluke	1–2.5 cm	Bile ducts	Mouth
Paragonimus westermani	Lung fluke	1.0 cm	Lungs	Mouth

Source of Infection, Intermediate Host or Vector	Most Common Clinical Symptoms	Laboratory Diagnosis	Therapeutic Agents	Remarks
Plerocercoid in fresh-water fish	Anemia very rare in the U.S.	Eggs in stool	Niclosamide Paromomycin Quinacrine	Prophylaxis by excreta disposal. Cook fish well
Cyst in pork	Usually none	Eggs and segments in stool; Scotch tape swab	Quinacrine Niclosamide Paromomycin	Uncommon in U.S. Frequent in Mexico, Central, South America
Eggs from feces, regurgitation of eggs	Intracranial pressure Epilepsy	Skin test, X ray of calcified cysts	Surgery	Uncommon in U.S. Autoinfection possible
Eggs from dog feces	Pressure symptoms in various organs	Skin, comp. fix., hemagglutination tests, X ray	Surgery	Uncommon in untraveled natives of U.S.
Cercaria in fresh water, from snail	Chronic dysentery, fibrosis of liver	Eggs in stool, rectal or liver biopsy	Stibophen Niridazole Astiban	Africa, South America. Common in Puerto Ricans
"	Urinary disturbances, hematuria	Eggs in urine, cystoscopy	Niridazole Astiban Stibophen	Africa, Middle East
"	Dysentery, hepatic fibrosis	Eggs in stool, liver biopsy	Antimony potassium tartrate Astiban Stibophen	China, Japan, Philippines, Celebes
Water nuts and vegetables	Diarrhea, edema, abdominal pain	Eggs in stool	Hexylresorcinol Tetrachlorethylene Bephenium hydroxynaphthoate	
Freshwater fish	Indigestion, diarrhea, hepatomegaly	Eggs in stool	Chloroquine Dehydroemetine Emetine	Usually in Asians
Freshwater crustaceans (crabs)	Hemoptysis, cough, abdominal pain, fever	Eggs in sputum and stool	Bithionol Chloroquine	Wandering worms in brain and other organs

guess what came to dinner?

	Common Name of Parasite or Disease	Length of Parasite	Site in Host	Portal of Entry
PROTOZOA				
Plasmodium vivax	Benign tertian malaria			
Plasmodium falciparum	Malignant tertian malaria	Intracellular	Liver parenchyma, red blood cells	Skin
Plasmodium malariae	Quartan malaria			
Plasmodium ovale				
Leishmania donovani	Visceral leish-maniasis, kala-azar	Intracellular 2 µ	Monocytes, P.M.N. endo-thelial cells	Skin
Leishmania tropica	Cutaneous leish-maniasis	"	In histiocytes of skin and mucosa	Skin
Leishmania braziliensis	Espundia, mucocu-taneous leish-maniasis	"	"	Skin
Trypanosoma gambiense	African sleeping sickness	14–33 µ	Lymph glands, bloodstream, brain	Skin
Trypanosoma rhodesiense				
Trypanosoma cruzi	South American trypanosomiasis	Intracellular stages Tryp. 20 µ	Tissues—heart Blood	Skin
Entamoeba histolytica	Intestinal ame-biasis	15–60 µ	Lumen and wall of large intestine	Mouth
" "	Amebic hepatitis Amebic liver abscess		Liver	Mouth

Source of Infection, Intermediate Host or Vector	Most Common Clinical Symptoms	Laboratory Diagnosis	Therapeutic Agents	Remarks
Anopheles mosquito Transfusions Drug addict syringe	Fever, chill, sweat, enlarged spleen Hemoglobinuria in "blackwater fever"	Repeated blood smears	Chloroquine Primaquine Sulfamethoxine Pyrimethamine Sulfadiazine Quinine Amodiaquine	Fever irregular in early disease. Incubation long after drug suppression. Drug-resistant strains
Phlebotomus (fly)	Fever, enlarged liver and spleen, leukopenia	Liver biopsy, sternal puncture, comp. fix, test, F.A.T.	Antimony sodium gluconate Pentamidine	Signs and symptoms resemble malaria
Phlebotomus	Chronic ulceration of exposed skin areas	Skin scrapings	Antimony sodium gluconate X ray, CO_2 snow	Immunity following lesion
Phlebotomus	Ulceration of naso-oral region	Scrape lesions	Antimony sodium gluconate Amphotericin B Cycloquanil pamoate	
Tsetse fly	Fever, rash, headache, spleen and liver enlarged	Blood smear, gland puncture, cerebrospinal fluid for trypanosomes	Pentamidine isethionate Suramin Melarsoprol Tryparsamide	Enlargement of posterior cervical lymph nodes, Winterbottom's sign
Kissing bug Triatomidae	Fever, spleen and liver enlarged Myocarditis	Blood smear, comp. fix., rat inoculation, F.A.T.	Bayer 2502 Primaquine	Unilateral periorbital edema, Megacolon, Megasophagus
Cysts in food and water, from feces	Mild to severe G.I. distress, dysentery	Cysts in cold stool, trophs in purged stool, serology	Diodoquin Paramomycin Dehydroemetine Chloroquine Emetine Tetracyclines Metronidazole	Consider possibility of hepatic infection
"	Enlarged tender liver, fever, leukocytosis	X ray, serology, cysts or trophs in stool	Metronidazole Dehydroemetine Chloroquine	Treat intestinal amebic infection

29

	Common Name of Parasite or Disease	Length of Parasite	Site in Host	Portal of Entry
PROTOZOA (*cont.*)				
Dientamoeba fragilis		5–12 μ	Large intestine	Mouth
Balantidium coli		50–100 μ	Large intestine	Mouth
Giardia lamblia	Flagellate diarrhea	11–18 μ	Upper small intestine	Mouth
Trichomonas vaginalis		10–30 μ	Vagina, prostate	Genitalia
Toxoplasma gondii	Toxoplasmosis	4–6 μ	All organs	Mouth
Pneumocystis carinii	Pneumonia	0.5–1.0 μ	Lungs	Respiratory
Naegleria sp.	Interstitial plasma cell pneumonia		Brain	Nose

granulomas

Granulomas are tumor-like masses that encase destroyed larva or parasitic eggs. They develop most often in the colon or rectal walls but can also be found in the lungs, liver, peritoneum, and uterus.

Source of Infection, Intermediate Host or Vector	Most Common Clinical Symptoms	Laboratory Diagnosis	Therapeutic Agents	Remarks
Stool (trophs)	Abdominal discomfort, diarrhea	Stool exam, trophs	Diodoquin Tetracyclines	Often asymptomatic
Stool (cyst)	Diarrhea, dysentery	Cysts and trophs in stool	Tetracyclines Diodoquin	Human and porcine sources
Cysts in food and water, from feces	Mild G.I. distress and diarrhea, weight loss	Cysts and trophs in stool	Metronidazole Quinacrine	More common in children than adults
Trophs in vaginal and prostatic secretion	Frothy vaginal discharge	Trophs in vaginal and prostatic fluid	Metronidazole	Treat both sexual partners
Congenital, Infected meat Oocysts in cat's stool	Chorioretinitis Hydrocephalus Convulsions Mimics infect. mono.	Biopsy, methylene blue dye test, comp. fix.	Pyrimethamine with trisulfapyrimidines	Cerebral calcification. Asymptomatic infections
Respiratory (?)	Pneumonia	Sputum exam, comp. fix. (?)	Pentamidine isethionate Pyrimethamine	Premature babies. Moribund adults
	C.N.S.		Amphotericin B.	Highly toxic

Source: Brown, Harold. *Basic Clinical Parasitology,* 4th ed., New York: Appleton-Century-Crofts, 1975, pages 4–11. Reprinted with permission.

nervousness

Parasitic metabolic wastes and toxic substances can serve as irritants to the central nervous system. Restlessness and anxiety are often the result of systemic parasite infestation.

sleep disturbances

Multiple awakenings during the night, particularly between 2 and 3 A.M., are possibly caused by the body's attempts to eliminate toxic wastes via the liver. According to Chinese medicine, these hours are governed by the liver. Sleep disturbances are also caused by nocturnal exits of certain parasites through the anus, creating intense discomfort and itching.

teeth grinding

Bruxism—abnormal grinding, clenching, and gnashing of the teeth—has been observed in cases of parasitic infection. These symptoms are most noticeable among sleeping children. Bruxism may be a nervous response to the internal foreign irritant. It is interesting to note that in the medical literature, the etiology of bruxism remains controversial.

chronic fatigue

Chronic fatigue symptoms include tiredness, flu-like complaints, apathy, depression, impaired concentration, and faulty memory. Parasites cause these physical, mental, and emotional symptoms through malnutrition resulting from malabsorption of proteins, carbohydrates, fats, and especially vitamins A and B_{12}.

immune dysfunction

Parasites depress immune system functioning by decreasing the secretion of immunoglobulin A (IgA). Their presence continuously stimulates the immune system response and over time can exhaust this vital defense system, leaving the body open to bacterial and viral infections.

summing up

Basically, parasites create damage to the host's body in six ways:

1. They destroy cells in the body faster than cells can be regenerated, thereby creating an imbalance that results in ulceration, perforation, or anemia.
2. They produce toxic substances that are harmful to the body. In cases of chronic infection, the body's immune response can be pushed into overdrive, producing elevated levels of eosinophils. Eosinophils are specialized white cells that normally combat any microscopic pathogen, but when their level is elevated, they themselves can cause tissue damage that results in pain and inflammation.
3. The presence of parasites irritates the tissues of the body, inducing an inflammatory reaction on the part of the host.
4. Some parasites invade the body by penetrating the skin, producing dermatitis. During their developmental stage, other parasites perforate and damage the intestinal lining.
5. The size and/or weight of the parasitic cysts, particularly if they are located in the brain, spinal cord, eye, heart, or bones, produces pressure effects on these organs. Obstruction, particularly of the intestine and pancreatic and bile ducts, can also occur.
6. The presence of parasites depresses immune system functioning while activating the immune response. This can eventually lead to immune system exhaustion.

Not every case of ill health can be blamed on parasites. But if symptoms persist and reoccur at regular intervals after you've been treated for some other diagnosed ailment, then parasites should be suspected. It is a good idea to keep track of your symptoms and look into the parasite connection with the assistance of an experienced health-care provider. The next chapters will help you to understand the parasite-based illnesses further.

3

guide to parasites

This chapter is a reference guide to the individual parasites. Because it is rather technical, you may not want to read it all the way through. You will find it useful to refer back to while reading later chapters. For the sake of not becoming too technical and academic, I have distilled the most pertinent clinical features of each parasite into a basic general description.

Experts calculate that there are approximately 300 different parasites existing in the United States today. The CDC, however, estimates the number to be much higher—even in the thousands. These parasites are biochemically complex creatures in their life histories, development, reproductive cycles, nutritional requirements, and disease manifestation. They are categorized according to structure, shape, function, and reproductive ability. These include microscopic organisms (protozoa); round-, pin-, and hookworms (nematoda); tapeworms (cestoda); and flukes (trematoda). The following is a discussion of each grouping and its outstanding characteristics.

protozoa

Making up approximately 70 percent of all parasites, protozoa are invisible to the naked eye. They are one-celled microscopic organisms, but don't let their size fool you. Certain protozoans, through their intensely rapid reproductive ability, can take over the intestinal tract of their host and from there go on to other organs and tissues. Some feed on red blood cells. Texas physician James Lewis aptly describes one such protozoan as "a microscopic vampire."[1] Some protozoa produce cysts—closed sacs in which they may be safely transported through food and water from one person to another. In the cyst state, protozoans are safe from destruction by human digestive juices. These one-celled "vampires," unlike their larger relatives, can actually destroy the tissues of their hosts. An estimated 7 million people across the U.S. have some form of protozoa living inside of them, according to experts. Common protozoa include *Giardia lamblia, Entamoeba histolytica, Cryptosporidum parvum, Blastocystis hominis,* and *Cyclospora cayetanensis.*

AMOEBA

Several varieties of amoeba found in humans are not considered disease-producing in normal individuals. Sometimes, however, virulent strains of otherwise nonpathogenic amoeba like *Entamoeba coli* and *Entamoeba hartmanni* can produce mild diarrhea and dysentery. Along with the *Acanthamoeba,* which can cause corneal ulcers in individuals who use tap water for sterilizing contact lenses, the amoeba listed here are the protozoans most commonly found to cause disease.

Entamoeba histolytica

Amebiasis, produced by *Entamoeba histolytica* infection, holds the dubious distinction of being the primary cause of death throughout the world today. Previous testing methods, which could not discern the parasite after seven weeks of infestation, helped make *E. histolytica* the *most commonly undetected* parasitic infection. During that time period, the parasite travels from the upper to the lower GI tract, then makes its way into the lymph nodes. There, it stops shedding and becomes undetectable. This drug-resistant protozoa penetrates the colon's nerve tissue and muscle. The ensuing antigens produce an autoimmune reaction, resulting in red inflammatory spots. With the colonic environment affected, the parasite can migrate into the liver and create abcesses. Shockingly, a number of deaths occur annually when unsuspecting individuals with parasitic liver abscesses undergo a liver biopsy. Death can occur within a few hours of the biopsy. Besides invading the liver, *E. histolytica* may also penetrate the brain and other body organs.

Steroids are also known to stimulate an existing *E. histolytica* infection. In fact, if the infection has been in a semi-dormant state, it will become active within a few days of using steroids. For this reason, it's vitally important that those persons receiving medical help for colon-related issues rule out an *E. histolytica* infection first before taking steroidal medication. This insidious parasite infects 10 percent of the world's population, causing 50 million cases of dysentery or liver abscesses and 100,000 deaths per year. (I personally suspect the infection rate to be much higher because of the difficulty in diagnosing *E. histolytica*.) *E. histolytica* is transmitted in cyst form from fecally contaminated food or water, infected food handlers, flies, or cockroaches. *Entamoeba histolytica* has a two-phase life cycle: the infective cyst and the latter trophozoite, which is motile and active. When cysts are ingested, they are first carried to the small intestine, where they are released as trophozoites to the colon. The trophozoite form of the parasite dwells primarily inside the bowel lumen, where it grows and multiplies. The incubation period varies from a few days up to three months. Changes in the host's resistance or the organism's pathogenicity can lead to tissue invasion. The trophozoite can then penetrate through the intestinal lining and invade the liver, lungs, brain, and heart.

Most cases of amebiasis do not produce clinical symptoms. Subclinical symptoms include right-upper quadrant pain, cramps, and occasional nausea and loose stools. In more serious cases, pronounced abdominal distension, dysentery, fever, and hepatitis may result. Extreme infection can cause abscesses in the liver, lungs, and even the brain. Chronic diarrhea, gas, and massive food and environmental allergies have all been reported when amoebas are found in the system. Amebic hepatitis can be mistaken for viral hepatitis; genital amebiasis for carcinoma; amebic colitis for ulcerative colitis; and amebiasis in the brain for brain tumor.

Endolimax nana

This amoeba cousin is a relatively new member of the bad-guy group of Protozoa, according to some researchers. It is the smallest of the intestinal amoebas, and the most convincing research of its underestimated virulence comes from Roger Wyburn-Mason, M.D., Ph.D., a British researcher who wrote *The Causation of Rheumatoid Disease and Many Human Cancers: A New Concept in Medicine* (*see* Suggested Reading List). Mason's book suggests that *Endolimax nana* is the cause of rheumatoid arthritis and a whole host of collagen-related diseases. This amoeba also lives in the lower bowel and can travel to other parts of the body. Besides the work of Dr. Wyburn-Mason, there have been relatively few reports of *Endolimax nana*'s pathogenicity. Some researchers now believe that Wyburn-Mason may have misidentified the amoeba-like organism; nevertheless, they agree that some kind of organism to which many individuals have become genetically susceptible causes rheumatoid arthritis.

Giardia lamblia

Like amoebas, giardia is transmitted in cyst form, which can live for up to six months under the fingernails. Giardia is recognized as one of the most infectious parasitic invaders, permeating entire households. Its cysts contaminate food and water via human or animal feces, such as dogs, cats, or parakeets. Tap water, mountain streams, and well water are prime sources of contamination. However, giardia is frequently spread in a number of other ways. According to a 1997 *Wall Street Journal* article, "There are a million modes of transmission . . . including sexual contact, poor personal hygiene, hand-to-mouth contact, and foodborne transmission by food handlers who don't wash their hands . . . Swimming pool outbreaks are common since giardia is resistant to chlorine."[2] It's no wonder the CDC reports approximately 2 million Americans are infected with giardia annually. And remember, these statistics are only for those given a diagnosis. Many individuals may be infected and not realize it.

After the cyst is swallowed and reaches the intestines, it reverts to the trophozoite stage. The hatched egg begins to replicate every 20 minutes, producing a full-fledged infection inside the human host within just 60 days. It adheres to the upper small intestine by means of a sucking disk and coats the lining of the intestinal mucosa, preventing digestion and assimilation of foods and causing a form of gastroenteritis. Following infection, symptoms develop after a one-to-three-week incubation period. Symptoms include diarrhea, bloat, foul-smelling gas, nausea, weight loss, heavy mucus, greasy stools, and abdominal cramping. Chills, low-grade fever, belching, and headache may also be present. After the initial episode, the symptoms may diminish, with intermittent diarrhea and constipation, abdominal distension, and foul-smelling gas persisting. The giardia can sometimes attach itself to the bile ducts of the liver, creating symptoms mimicking gallbladder disease. Once giardia has worked its way into the bile ducts and gallbladder, a liver/gallbladder flush may be needed to expel the eggs into the GI tract and upper duodenum, where they can be eradicated. (It's important to note that giardia is extremely determined. If there is even just one giardia cyst remaining, it will hatch and replicate, throwing the human host once again into infection 60 days after treatment.)

Damage to the intestinal villi from the giardia can persist long after the infection is controlled. Problems like chronic iron deficiency, anemia, deficiencies of vitamins A and B_{12}, low serum calcium, lack of folic acid, fat malabsorption, and lactose intolerance occur with prolonged infection. Chronic fatigue and depression are symptomatic of long-standing giardiasis. Individuals appear to be more at risk if they have type A blood, lack of hydrochloric acid, or have a history of *Candida albicans*. (Giardia infection can accelerate transit time and subsequently force undigested particles into the colon, where they can nourish organisms such as *Candida albicans*.) In small children and the elderly, severe dehydration caused by diarrhea, and vomiting can be fatal. In children, giardia can be misdiagnosed as celiac disease or failure-to-thrive syndrome.

Cryptosporidium parvum

Once thought as only existing in immune-compromised persons, the microscopic *Cryptosporidium parvum* has quickly become the principal cause of infectious diarrhea in preschool children. And, much like giardia, cryptosporidium is found in day-care centers, where it is directly related to diaper-changing practices. Agricultural runoffs and sewage leaks have been known to carry this pathogenic parasite into municipal water supplies. First recognized in baby calves, cryptosporidium has emerged as a global public health problem with epidemic proportions in such "diverse settings as dairy farms, urban slums in developing countries, and water-borne outbreaks in developed countries," according to a 1996 article in *Parasitology Today*.[3] The parasite penetrates healthy cells and thrives there for seven days. Afterward it leaves, destroying the cell it once hosted. An individual may not exhibit any symptoms except during the parasite's migratory period. At that point, the intestinal lining may become inflamed, producing alternating bouts of diarrhea and constipation. Malabsorption, increased permeability, and a leaky gut syndrome may also ensue, causing various food allergies, colitis, and bowel toxicities.

Blastocystis hominis

First classified as a non-pathogenic yeast, blastocystis is now recognized by some researchers as a protozoan. The organism does not have the cyst and trophozoite stages of a typical protozoan, however. Blastocystis infects intestines in the region where the small intestine meets the colon. When the organism is found in great enough numbers in the intestinal tract, its host often complains of nausea, gas, abdominal pain, diarrhea, and malaise. A 1996 report by Dr. Omar Amin reported of the "44 symptomatic patients infected with B. hominis, 18 had very heavy infections. Sixteen of these people had been travelers to the subcontinent of India."[4] And of the tested subjects, some had unresolved infections despite two years of treatment. At the Great Smokies Diagnostic Laboratory (see page 144), this parasite is one of the most commonly detected in stool samples.

Cyclospora cayetanensis

After the parasite Cyclospora cayetanenis caused its first reported outbreak in 1994, it formed a stronghold in the U.S. The parasite can cause days, sometimes weeks, of diarrhea, weight loss, fatigue, and gastrointestinal distress. In 1996 almost 1,000 fell ill to an outbreak traced to cyclospora-contaminated raspberries imported from Guatemala. Also in 1997, cyclospora contaminated a wedding party in wealthy Westchester County, New York. The vehicle of the infection was imported raspberries from Guatemala and Chile. Then in 1998 a group of Texas business executives became ill after a luncheon in Houston: At least six were infected with the cyclospora parasite.[5] According to a 1996 report by Dr. Omar Amin, vital connections exist between parasite-infected household contacts and increased risk of parasitic infections. He observed a relationship between current and earlier parasitic infections. Dr. Amin also implicated foreign travel as a contributing factor to the prevalence of infection. With fecal samples taken from 5,250 patients from 49 states, three Canadian provinces, and five foreign countries, cyclospora was found in 225 patients, revealing females as being 2.5 times more frequently infected than males. Of the infected patients, 128 experienced gastrointestinal symptoms, such as bloating, diarrhea, flatulence, cramps, constipation, fatigue, and allergies. These infected patients traveled most frequently to Mexico and Europe. Some 6 percent of these patients lived with infected household contacts and 11 percent of them had previous parasitic infections with various protozoans or worms.

Trichomonas vaginalis

Trichomonas vaginalis, found only in trophozoite form, is a sexually transmitted organism. However, some infections are probably passed through sauna benches, towels, toilet seats, and therapeutic mud and water baths.

Trichomonas can exist in the urethra, in the endocervical and urethral glands, or in the prostate without causing inflammation. Approximately 25 percent of men and approximately 40 percent of women can be host to the organism without showing symptoms. Foul-smelling cheesy vaginal discharge, painful urination, frequent urination, and small vaginal lesions are symptomatic. This organism is capable of producing inflammatory changes on the bladder, urethra, and mucosal surfaces of the vagina.

Trichomoniasis is commonly recognized as a female problem but should also be considered as a possible cause of problems with the male reproductive tract. Males who suffer from prostate infections or painful urination would do well to consider the possibility of trichomonas infection. Non-specific urinary complaints may have their roots in trichomonas because it is passed between sexual partners.

Toxoplasma gondii

Humans can acquire toxoplasmosis from cats, because the cysts of *Toxoplasma gondii* are passed through their feces. These cysts become infectious within three to four days and remain viable for up to eighteen months. Breathing dust containing infectious eggs is another pathway for transmission. Eating undercooked or improperly cooked meat (such as beef, pork, lamb, and rabbit) is another source of infection. Infection can also be acquired through organ transplants or congenitally.

Toxoplasmosis is a prime example of an asymptomatic disease. It is estimated that up to 50 percent of the adult population in America may be carrying a latent infection. In acute forms of the infection, symptoms resemble mononucleosis and include chills, fever, headache, and fatigue. Chronic-phase symptoms include hepatitis, swollen lymph glands, and, in some cases, blindness. Because of the lymph involvement, toxoplasmosis can be misdiagnosed as Hodgkin's disease. In non-immune pregnant women during the first trimester, toxoplasma can cross the placenta barrier, resulting in blindness, mental retardation, and even death to the unborn child. In immunosuppressed individuals, such as those with AIDS, toxoplasmosis is considered an opportunistic infection and affects the central nervous system, brain, lungs, and heart. Other symptoms of an active infection are encephalitis, paralysis on one side of the body, delusional behavior, and intense headaches that are unresponsive to painkillers.

Cryptosporidium muris

Transmitted via contaminated ground water, farm animals, and the fecal-oral route, *Cryptosporidium muris,* like giardia, is found in day-care centers and is directly related to diaper-changing practices. In healthy patients, the infection is usually mild and of short duration. Symptoms include abdominal discomfort, weight loss, fever, and nausea. Long known to cause diarrhea in animals, these organisms have now been identified as a major cause of diarrhea in humans. In immunocompromised individuals, particularly those with AIDS, *Cryptosporidium muris* has a life-threatening potential because it can cause severe dehydration and electrolyte imbalances.

Pneumocystis carinii

Acquired by the respiratory route, spores from this widespread organism are inhaled into the body. The trophozoites attach themselves to pulmonary tissue cells. Symptoms include dry cough, fever, weight loss, fatigue, night sweats, and difficulty breathing. This amoeba creates a kind of pneumonia that often causes death by asphyxiation in immunocompromised patients and premature babies.

Plasmodium malariae, Plasmodium ovale, Plasmodium vivax, Plasmodium falciparum

Four kinds of plasmodium, one-celled protozoans, infect humans. Because they cause malaria, these protozoa may be the most widely recognized.

There are several types of malaria, all transmitted by the bite of an infected anopheles mosquito.

Once established, the organism invades the red blood cells and destroys them. Malaria can take from four weeks to several months to develop. This is why it is essential to continue protective medication for at least a month after leaving an endemic area. Initially, patients exhibit high fever, shaking, chills, and other flu-like symptoms. Attacks of chills, high fever, and severe sweating can occur every 48 or 72 hours. Unexplained, recurring fever, malaise, headache, anemia, and enlarged liver and spleen are the most common chronic symptoms. Death can result from multi-system failure, including renal failure and ruptured spleen.

Malaria can be of the acute malignant type or the chronic relapsing type. Malaria is most commonly found in Africa, South America, and Southeast Asia. Recent cases have been reported in New Jersey and Rhode Island, with an annual outbreak reported in San Diego.

Leishmania donovani, Leishmania tropica, Leishmania braziliensis

These parasitic protozoans enter their hosts through the skin and grow to approximately 2 microns (roughly .000078 inches). Leishmaniasis, the parasitic disease found in the troops returning from Operation Desert Storm, is transmitted by sand flies. There are two types of disease manifestations: One consists of frequently ulcerated skin or mucosal lesions; the other, more serious one infects the internal organs, like the lymph nodes, liver, bone marrow, and spleen. This disease is most commonly found in Africa, Latin America, India, and the Middle East.

nematoda

This section will introduce you to the larger parasites, commonly known as worms. While the protozoans are only single-celled, these creatures are multicellular. The adult worms multiply by producing eggs called ova or larvae. The eggs usually become infectious in soil or in an intermediate host before humans are infected. It is interesting to note that unless the worm infestation is heavy, many individuals do not show signs of disease. While it may be unpleasant to consider, it is true that the human host can coexist quite comfortably with a few worms, unless they reproduce in great numbers and create organ obstruction.

According to Dr. Hazel Parcells, a leading parasite and alternative medicine expert, worms are "the most toxic agents in the human body . . . and one of the primary underlying causes of disease." Experts support her statement, claiming some type of worm is already in the intestines of over 75 percent of the world's population.

ROUNDWORM (*Ascaris lumbricoides*)

The most common intestinal parasite in the world is the large roundworm known as the *Ascaris lumbricoides*. About 1 billion people are infected with ascaris. Due to their oral tendencies, children are very prone to roundworm. The worm resembles the common earthworm in appearance and is spread directly to humans from soil or food contaminated with human feces. It is found worldwide and is more common in tropical and subtropical areas, especially in Asia because of the use there of night soil (human excrement) as fertilizer.

Once the worms develop in the human system, they can pass through the liver and lungs, where they create severe tissue irritation and allergic reactions. Adult worms can travel through the body and end up in the liver, heart, and lungs. They can create intestinal obstruction when present in large enough numbers. Symptoms in children include nervousness, colic, poor appetite, failure to thrive, allergic reactions, coughing, and wheezing. Malnutrition in children is also characteristic of heavy ascaris infection because the worms compete for food. Ascaris inhibits absorption of proteins, fats, and carbohydrates. Adults can exhibit vague abdominal pain, edema (abnormal accumulation of fluid) of the lips, allergic reactions, insomnia, anorexia, and weight loss.

HOOKWORM (*Necator americanus, Ancylostoma duodenal*)

Hookworm larvae are found in warm moist soil. They enter the body by penetrating the skin and are often found in people who frequently go barefoot. Hookworms travel through the bloodstream to the lungs, into the alve-oli, and up the trachea to the throat, where they are swallowed and end up in their final habitat, the small intestine, in about seven weeks. When the larvae pass through the lungs, bronchitis may develop. The teeth-like hooks of the larvae attach to the intestinal mucosa and rob the body of large amounts of blood. Found worldwide in warm, moist tropical areas, hook-worms in the United States are most prevalent in the southeastern part of the country.

The first symptom of hookworm infection is itchy patches of skin, pim-ples and/or blisters known as ground itch (dew itch). Other symptoms in-clude itching at entry site, nausea, dizziness, pneumonitis, anorexia, weight loss, and anemia. These worms can live up to fifteen years in the human body.

PINWORM (*Enterobius vermicularis*)

The most common of all the worms in the United States, the pinworm is most prevalent in children. Transmission occurs through contaminated food, water, and house dust as well as human-to-human contact. The adult female pinworm moves outside the anus to lay eggs. These eggs are often transferred by a child's fingers from the itching anal area to the mouth. Children can easily transmit the worms to the entire family through the bathtub, toilet seat, and bedclothes.

Perianal itching is the most classic pinworm symptom. But these little quarter-inch mobile worms that resemble threads have been connected to an enormous range of neurological and behavioral symptoms. Pediatrician Leo Litter, in a ten-year study of over 2,000 cases of children with pin-worms, documented seemingly unrelated symptoms that previously had not been associated with this parasitic infection. Some of the more unusual symptoms include abnormal electroencephalograms (EEGs)—sometimes resembling those in cases of brain tumor—epilepsy, hyperactivity, and vi-sion problems. (Dr. Litter's tips are listed on page 110. If you have children or teach, please read them.)

STRONGYLOIDES *(Stronglyoides stercoralis)*

This nematode is unique because the mature adult can reproduce entirely in the human host or grow into a free-living worm in soil. Strongyloides produce autoinfection in the host and can remain in the body for more than thirty years. Found in Southeast Asia and the southeastern part of the United States, this parasite is extremely difficult to diagnose. The infection is transmitted when larvae penetrate the human through the skin, pores, or hair follicles. Most commonly, invasion occurs between the toes or at the bottom of the foot. The larvae then reach maturity in the intestines. When the larvae invade tissue (primarily the intestinal wall and lung), a condition known as disseminated strongyloides develops; this condition can be fatal.

Abdominal bloating and gastrointestinal problems (including diarrhea and greasy stools) are the primary symptoms. Infections have been known to last up to thirty-six years, with the predominant symptoms being nausea, bloating, diarrhea, and pulmonary disorders. This parasitic condition is often found in AIDS victims.

TRICHINELLA *(Trichinella spiralis)*

Just about any symptom known to man can be caused by the various stages of trichinosis infection, which can masquerade as at least fifty more familiar diseases ranging from flu to generalized and specific aches and pains. Most roundworms are transmitted through soil contaminated by feces, but the small spiral-shaped trichinella found in pork is the exception. These tiny roundworms can become enclosed in a cyst inside the muscles of bears, walruses, and pigs. If pork is eaten and not thoroughly cooked, the cysts are dissolved by the host's digestive juices, and the worms mature and travel to the muscles, where they become encased. Eventually the worms can burrow into the larynx, chest, diaphragm, abdomen, jaws, and upper arms. Then they calcify, causing severe muscle soreness and fever.

The symptoms of trichinosis change according to the progress the trichinella make through the body. During the first week of infection, acute diarrhea, nausea, vomiting, and colic occur as the larvae penetrate the first part of the small intestine. Then, when the larvae migrate to muscle tissue, about two to four weeks after the infected meat was eaten, the most classical symptom, severe muscle pain, is experienced. When the larvae finally encyst themselves in muscle fiber, extreme dehydration and toxic edema can be caused. Edema of the lips, face, or eyelids, difficulty in breathing or speaking, chewing problems, enlarged lymph glands, meningitis, and encephalitis can take place. Brain damage, pneumonia, pleurisy, and nephritis are further complications of this disease.

ANISAKINE LARVAE

Anisakid worms have a two-host life cycle: The adult lives in sea mammals, and the infected larval stages appear in fish like Pacific salmon, Pacific rockfish (red snapper), herring, cod, and haddock. Humans become infected by consuming raw, pickled, or smoked herring, or by eating undercooked fish—a common occurrence when relying on the microwave. Symptoms include appendicitis, Crohn's disease, and intestinal inflammation. Sometimes the worms have to be surgically removed because of perforation.

DOG AND CAT ROUNDWORM
(*Toxocara canis, toxocara cati*)

Toxocara canis and *Toxocara cati* are dog and cat roundworms that cause a disease called visceral larva migrans in humans, mainly children. Food, water, and soil contaminated with roundworm eggs are the most common routes of infection. Children are the most common victims of this malady because of their hand-to-mouth habits and because their play areas may be contaminated by roundworm eggs from dogs and cats.

The human is not a viable host for the mature dog or cat worm, but the immature form causes visceral larva migrans. When the larvae hatch, they travel to various parts of the body like the lungs, liver, brain, or eyes. They cause enlarged liver, abdominal pain, and often pneumonitis. A high eosinophil count as well as anemia are typical of this problem.

FILARIA (*Wuchereria bancrofti, Brugia malayi, Onchocerca volvulus, Loa loa, Mansonella streptocerca, Mansonella perstans, Mansonella ozzardi*)

Including dog heartworm, there are eight species of filariae known to infect people. Transmitted by bloodsucking insects and flies, the filariae are microscopic roundworms that cause diseases endemic to tropical Africa, Southeast Asia, and the South Pacific. The lymphatic filariae—*Wuchereria bancrofti* and *Brugia malayi*—invade the bloodstream and lymphatics with pronounced effects ranging from simple fever and lymph node infection to deformities like elephantiasis of the legs, arms, scrotum, and breasts. *Onchocerca volvulus* causes dermatitis, subcutaneous nodules, and eye lesions. In some areas of West Africa, almost 30 percent of all adults are blind because of this parasite. Onchocerciasis is known as "river blindness" because the disease occurs in Africa near rivers where the vector flies breed. Other filarial infections include *Loa loa*, characterized by temporary loss of vision and transient swellings. All three species of the *Mansonella* filariae cause a type of itching dermatitis.

DOG HEARTWORM (*Dirofilaria immitis*)

The most endemic areas in the United States for human dog heartworm infection are the Mississippi River Valley and the Atlantic and Gulf Coasts. Man is not a viable host for the fully mature worm; it is the heartworm larvae that invade man. The parasite, which is transmitted by an infected mosquito, usually remains in subcutaneous tissue. The larvae rarely complete their life cycle, but if they do, they migrate to the lung, where they become localized in a coin-like lesion. The symptoms are generally mild, with an occasional cough. The major problem is that on an X ray the lesion can be mistaken for cancer, leading to unnecessary surgery.

cestoda

Among the oldest known parasites, tapeworms are considered humanity's largest intestinal inhabitant. Reportedly, they can reach lengths of up to 36 inches or more. They each have a scolex, or head, that attaches to the intestinal wall. As long as the head remains attached to the intestinal mucosa, a new worm can grow from it. Tapeworms do not contain digestive tracts but get their nourishment by absorbing partially digested substances from the host. They are whitish in color, flat, and ribbon-like, with a covering that is a transparent skin-like layer.

BEEF TAPEWORM (*Taenia saginata*)

Beef tapeworm can be ingested from raw or undercooked beef (rare or medium rare). Despite its size, several feet long, the beef tapeworm does not produce marked symptoms. It is composed of 1,000-to-2,000-segment strands. The segment known as the proglottid, which contains both male and female reproductive organs, bears the eggs. Tapeworms thrive on the diet of the host for their carbohydrates but utilize the tissues of the host for proteins.

Beef tapeworms have a life span in the intestine of twenty to twenty-five years. Usually, only one worm at a time infects the system. Because the worm's presence produces few symptoms, it is rather surprising when the proglottids move out of the anus unexpectedly as they sometimes do. Symptoms such as diarrhea, abdominal cramping, nervousness, nausea, and loss of appetite are possible.

PORK TAPEWORM (*Taenia solium*)

Pork tapeworm is similar to beef tapeworm but is shorter, with less than 1,000 proglottids. Pork tapeworm infects man through the eating of infested undercooked pork such as fresh or smoked ham or sausage. Unlike the beef tapeworm, pork tapeworm infection is usually caused by multiple worms rather than just one. The larva stage develops in the muscle, spreads through the central nervous system into other tissues and organs, and finally hooks onto the upper small intestine.

Pork tapeworm causes great harm to the human host when the immature larvae invade the muscles, heart, eyes, or brain. The larval migration of pork tapeworm represents the most dangerous infection of all the tapeworms. In the brain, the worms can create a condition known as cysticercosis, which can produce seizures and brain deterioration and often is misdiagnosed as epilepsy.

FISH TAPEWORM (*Diphyllobothrium latum*)

The largest parasite found in humans, a fish tapeworm has up to 4,000 proglottids (the worm's primary body) and may even deposit over 1,000,000 eggs daily in its human host. It is commonly found in Scandinavia, Russia, Japan, Australia, the Great Lakes, Canada, and Alaska. It can be contracted by eating raw or lightly cooked freshwater or certain migratory species of fish, such as Alaskan salmon, perch, pike, pickerel, and American turbot. In the intestine, fish tapeworm can consume 80 to 100 percent of the host's vitamin B_{12}. A striking vitamin B_{12} deficiency or pernicious anemia is the most debilitating effect. Digestive disturbances—including pain and fullness in the upper abdomen, nausea, and anorexia—are common symptoms.

DOG TAPEWORM (*Dipylidium caninum*)

Dog tapeworm is transmitted by infected dog fleas. Of all human hosts, children are the most common. By kissing dogs or by having the dogs "kiss" them, children may accidentally swallow an infected dog flea. Called the "pumpkinseed tapeworm," the first hint of its infection may be finding pumpkin-seed–like particles in the stool of the child or in his or her undergarments. These particles are actually the egg-bearing segments (proglottids) of the tapeworm. After the flea is swallowed, the larva is liberated, and in twenty days, the worm reaches maturity. Symptoms are vague but include restlessness and persistent diarrhea.

trematoda

Trematoda are leaf-shaped flatworms also known as flukes. They are para-sitic during nearly all of their life cycle forms. The cycle begins when larvae are released into freshwater by infected snails. The free-swimming larvae can then directly penetrate the skin of the human host or are ingested after encycsting in or on various edible vegetation, fish, or crustaceans.

BLOOD FLUKE (*Schistosoma japonicum, Schistosoma mansoni, Schistosoma haematobium*)

There are three primary species of blood flukes, or schistosomes, that cause disease. One of the three types of resulting diseases, *Schistosomiasis man-soni,* occurs in Africa, the Eastern Mediterranean, the Caribbean, and South America. Another, *Schistosomiasis japonicum,* is found in Asia. The third, *Schistosomiasis haematobium,* is found in Egypt. Freshwater snails play intermediate host in the life cycle development of these blood flukes. The snails release larvae into water, where the larvae can directly penetrate the skin of swimmers or bathers in contaminated rivers or streams.

The parasite burrows into the skin and is carried through the blood-stream to the veins of the liver, intestines, or bladder. In two forms of schis-tosomiasis, inflammation begins when the worms lodge in the lining of the intestine or liver. In another form, the bladder and urinary tract can become fatally infected by worms lodged in the walls of the bladder.

LIVER FLUKE (*Clonorchis sinensis*)

Common in Asia and Hawaii, the liver fluke is transmitted through the in-gestion of raw, dried, salted, pickled, or undercooked fish. Snails, carp, and forty additional species of fish have been known to be intermediate hosts to this fluke. In the human, it inhabits the bile ducts of the liver, causing the liver to become enlarged and tender. It also causes inflammation, chills, fever, jaundice, and a type of hepatitis.

ORIENTAL LUNG FLUKE (*Paragonimus westermani*)

Found in the Far East, the lung fluke enters the body via infected crabs and crayfish that have been insufficiently cooked or eaten raw. The adult worms go to the lungs and even the brain, where seizures similar to epilepsy can occur. Symptoms include an occasionally mild cough and a peculiar blood-stained, brown, rusty sputum when a victim wakes. The lung fluke can perforate lung tissue and deplete oxygen supplies to the entire bloodstream. Symptoms often resemble those of pulmonary tuberculosis.

SHEEP LIVER FLUKE (*Fasciola hepatica*)

Cases of this fluke have been reported in Central and South America, parts of Africa, Asia, and Australia. Infection is usually acquired from eating worm larvae encysted on a aquatic vegetation such as watercress. Worms migrate to the liver and bile ducts, where they produce right-upper-quadrant abdominal pain, liver abscesses, and fibrosis.

INTESTINAL FLUKE (*Fasciolopsis buski*)

Human infections occur mainly in Southeast Asia. Transmission occurs when individuals bite into the unpeeled outer skin of plants that harbor encycsted larvae. Such plants can include water chestnuts, bamboo shoots, and lotus plant roots. Adult flukes live in the duodenum (the shortest, widest portion of the small intestine) and jejunum (connecting the duodenum and the ileum, which opens into the large intestine), where they cause ulceration. Symptoms include diarrhea, nausea, vomiting, abdominal pain, and facial and abdominal edema.

As you have learned, parasites are responsible for an enormous panorama of worldwide human health problems. These organisms are very well equipped to gain access to the human body, where they can reproduce through unique life cycle processes that evade our body's defenses. In the next chapters we will examine the invaders' major portals of entry.

4

the water and
food connection

Food and water are the most common sources of parasite-based illness. Since most of us eat three times a day and drink water frequently throughout the day, our exposure to these sources is constant. Tap water has been found to be contaminated with parasitic organisms. Both plant and animal foods carry parasites, and cleaning and cooking methods often don't destroy them before ingestion. Today, because of environmental pollution, we all must pay careful attention to the purity of our water and the cleanliness of our food.

And with dining out being such a favorite American pastime, there's even more reason for us to be vigilant. The CDC cites food as the catalyst behind 80 percent of the pathogenic outbreaks in the U.S. Most are linked to restaurants and delis where less than sanitary conditions exist—from the food preparation and storage to the utensils and servers' hands. Clearly, it's time for us all to take a second look at our water and food.

the water connection

Studies indicate contaminated water accounts for nearly 1,000 deaths annually in the U.S. as well as more than a million gastrointestinal maladies.

A perfect example occurred in 1996 when a couple threw a high school graduation party for their daughter. The festive occasion took a dark turn as over 100 of their guests fell ill. Bacteria from the catering company's water made its way into the food. The culprits, salmonella and a rare tropical bug, triggered a malicious diarrhea and nausea.[1]

Obviously, this is not an isolated incident. Such waterborne illnesses continue to be on the rise. Unfortunately many of us shrug off the warning signs as the flu or even food poisoning. Seldom do we see a doctor or get properly tested for water-related diseases. And that can prove to be deadly, especially for senior citizens, pregnant women, or people with compromised immune systems. It's imperative that these individuals heed the warning issued by the CDC for the past five years: Boil your water no matter what the source.

Checking the source is still, however, critically important because 86 percent of small water systems have violated drinking water regulations. According to Erik Olson of the Natural Resources Defense Council, ". . . we have water systems that are repeat, significant violators and they're getting off scot-free." Part of the problem lies in enforcement. The EPA directed only a mere 1 percent of their $449 million 1998 enforcement budget for guaranteeing that we have good-quality water.

In infested waters, mosquitoes and flies can pick up eggs and cysts and transmit them to humans. Sewage sites are also prime parasite reservoirs. Scuba divers and recreational swimmers need to be concerned about the parasite population in freshwater lakes, ponds, and rivers. Divers can become infected with giardia and *Entamoeba histolytica*. In 1983, the scuba divers of New York City who work for the police and fire department had a 22-percent incidence of protozoan infection, probably from the polluted Hudson and East rivers, where more than 188 million gallons of sewage is dumped on a daily basis.[2]

Water is a main avenue for the spread of giardiasis in this country and abroad. For the past several years, the Centers for Disease Control has reported that the giardia organism is the most prevalent cause of water-borne disease in America. According to the Environmental Protection Agency, outbreaks in treated municipal water are doubling every five years. Giardiasis symptoms include diarrhea, bloating, foul gas, nausea, cramping, and intestinal irritation. Symptoms may last for several weeks or months and can even linger on in periodic episodes for years. The exact number of cases in this country remains unknown, since reporting is not required. Because of the number of ignored or misdiagnosed conditions (giardiasis is often diagnosed as irritable bowel syndrome and chronic fatigue), many researchers suspect the true number of giardiasis cases is astronomical.

Estimates are that 90 percent of the documented cases of water-borne giardia are coming from surface water that has become contaminated by wild animal feces, such as feces from beaver, muskrat, bear, possum, and raccoon. A few giardia cases have been connected to contaminated water from shallow wells. Giardia used to be referred to as "beaver fever," as it was once thought the beaver was the only animal that harbored the cyst. Breakdowns in municipal water systems, particularly in the more mountainous areas of this country, are a major cause of the rise of giardia in America today. Many of these water supplies are supported by reservoirs that rely on backcountry streams and lakes.

GIARDIA

Giardia has been found in the waters of the Cascade, Sierra, Rocky, Pacific Northwest, and Appalachian mountains. It has also been found in back streams feeding the municipal water supply of San Francisco. The most widely reported national outbreaks have occurred in Aspen, Colorado; Pittsfield, Massachusetts; Portland, Oregon; Berlin, New Hampshire; Scranton, Pennsylvania; Camas, Washington; and upper New York State. In Rome, New York, approximately 5,000 people became sick from giardia-infected water, resulting in the most serious recent outbreak of giardia in this country. The September–October 1991 issue of *In Health* reports that Pennsylvania leads the country in cases of water-borne disease. Between 1979 and 1990, 15,508 cases of giardia were reported in Pennsylvania. Who knows how many more cases occurred there but were misdiagnosed and not reported? This same article also reports dramatic increases in giardia in New York State, Wisconsin, Washington State, and Vermont, where giardia is now the leading water-borne disease.[3]

With the increasing development of recreational areas along reservoirs that supply public drinking water, the problem may be growing. People who are infected and use these recreational facilities for boating, fishing, or swimming may further contaminate what comes out of our faucets.

Giardia is a tiny organism. About 8,000 trophozoites can fit on the head of a pin. Without a microscope, a person cannot tell if water is infected. No matter how pristine the water source may seem, isolated and remote streams, rivers, and lakes can become contaminated with animal waste. Therefore, all hikers, campers, bikers, hunters, and swimmers should always refrain from drinking wilderness water unless it is properly treated.

Giardia cysts are very hearty and can exist up to three months in cold or tepid water. They are not always killed by chlorination, the most common chemical treatment used for water purification in municipal water supplies. They can be destroyed by iodine-based compounds. However, if the water temperature is close to freezing or contains a great deal of organic material, the amount of iodine necessary to inactivate the cysts makes the water unpalatable. Two commercially available water purification products that are iodine-based and designed for travelers, backpackers, hikers, and campers are Globaline and Polar Pure. Iodine has additional drawbacks. It can cause accidental poisoning and may be contraindicated in sensitive or allergic individuals.

It seems that boiling and filtration are the only surefire ways to kill giardia. At sea level, the water must be brought to a rolling boil and maintained there for at least ten minutes. At higher elevations, boil an additional five minutes. A rolling boil will also kill other protozoans and bacteria. Possibly the most reliable method of purification is through a mechanical filter. The filter must be fine enough to filter out the giardia cyst. The filter size should be no greater than 3 microns (a micron equals one millionth of a meter) because the giardia cyst is approximately 5 microns in size. (See Chapter Nine for specific filter recommendations.)

It is important to realize that giardiasis can also occur by eating vegetables or fruits that have been washed with contaminated water. Unpeeled or uncooked vegetables and fruit should be avoided in areas where giardia is suspect. This precaution, which is generally given to travelers abroad, needs to be observed here in the United States because of the increasing prevalence of outbreaks of giardia.

guess what came to dinner?

AMOEBA

Another one-celled organism, the amoeba, is also water-borne. The pathogenic form of this microorganism, *Entamoeba histolytica,* causes dysentery, diarrhea, cramping, and a host of other unpleasant symptoms. Only a few amebic cysts ingested from a glass of water are necessary to cause infection. Amebic cysts resist iodine and chlorine purification when the concentrations of these chemicals are too low.

Probably the most publicized outbreak of water-borne disease in this country occurred in Chicago around the time of the 1933 World's Fair. The infection (a form of amebic dysentery) was traced to the plumbing in a hotel, where a cross-connection had been made between the water pipes and sewage system in an attempt to repair a broken pipe. With the flushing of every toilet, sewage backed up into the drinking water system. About 1,400 people became infected, and 100 people died.[4]

The acanthamoeba is another type of amoeba found in tap water. It has been known to cause severe eye infections among contact lens wearers who wash their contact lenses in tap water without further disinfection. This infection, *Acanthamoeba keratitis,*[5] causes pain and inflammation around the cornea. In severe cases, the infection can progress, producing a corneal ulcer and in some cases necessitating corneal transplant. While relatively few cases have been reported, *Acanthamoeba keratitis* may be misdiagnosed for other conditions. To avoid ancanthamoeba, all contact lens wearers should use commercially prepared lens cleansing and disinfecting solutions.

LARGER PARASITES

Water can also contain the eggs and larvae of larger parasites like ascaris, hookworm, and the blood flukes or schistosomes. Particular care should be taken when traveling abroad, not only with drinking water, but with activities like swimming, bathing, rafting, canoeing, boating, and fishing, where direct skin contact can lead to penetration by the blood fluke. Schistosomiasis is a danger in Asia, Africa, and the Middle East, particularly Egypt. This parasitic infection has been reported in American travelers, for example, who river-rafted in African water.[6]

56

In this country, some environmentalists see the prevalence of giardia and the incidence of other water-borne parasites as an urgent call to action for other toxic problems endemic to our water supplies. With ever-increasing outbreaks of this infection, communities will be forced to update antiquated water systems that not only breed giardia but deliver bacteria, viruses, lead, and other contaminants to drinking water. The Environmental Protection Agency has set new standards for municipal drinking water systems that draw their water from surface supplies like reservoirs, lakes, streams, and ponds. Guidelines for the new Surface Water Treatment Rule include reducing levels of giardia, as well as other disease-producing viruses and bacteria, to practically zero.

the food connection

According to statistics from the Centers for Disease Control, each year approximately 9,000 in the U.S. die from contaminated food and scores of others fall seriously ill. Not only are the well-publicized bacteria *E. coli* and salmonella thwarting our health, but they are apparently mutating in an effort to generate resistant genes. *E. coli* 0157:H7 alone, per the CDC, is responsible for 250 deaths and 20,000 illnesses, including acute kidney failure in children.

When parasites are in food, they are almost always transmitted because of improper cooking practices—either too little cooking or none at all. While it is true that the majority of food-borne infections come from animal sources, like pork, beef, lamb, fish, and seafood, vegetarians are not immune. Many plant foods, such as watercress, bamboo shoots, water chestnuts, and lotus roots, may contain parasites in some form. Leafy vegetables, notably lettuce, parsley, and celery, can become contaminated by fertilizers made from human waste in some countries. For this reason, imported produce from Mexico and other Latin American countries should be thoroughly washed using the Clorox bath described in Chapter Nine.

guess what came to dinner?

PORK

The best-known illness caused by a food-borne parasite is undoubtedly trichinosis from pork. Caused by the *Trichinella spiralis* organism, trichinosis can also result from eating undercooked rabbit, wild boar, exotic meats like fox and polar bear, or jerky made from these meats. Polar bear meat infected with trichinella was finally determined to have been the mysterious cause of death in 1897 of three Arctic explorers; thus ended a sixty-year-old mystery.[7]

Trichinosis in this country usually comes from eating undercooked pork. Trichinosis is first transmitted to pigs when they are fed uncooked garbage or when infested rodents, like mice or rats, invade the hogs' feeding areas. A person becomes a host when, upon eating insufficiently cooked pork, the encysted larvae hatch in the intestines and migrate to encyst in muscles. Trichinosis is characterized by a flu-like illness and severe muscle aches and pains, mimicking at least fifty other illnesses.

While rare or undercooked pork can produce trichinosis, raw, rare, or undercooked pork, smoked ham, and sausage can also carry pork tapeworm infection. The latter is particularly harmful to the body if the pork tapeworm eggs migrate to the brain, where they will hatch into larvae and create cysticercosis, a condition that produces dementia, epilepsy, and sometimes death. The round cyst-like organisms (cysticerci) in the meat make it taste sweeter. Infected pork, because it tastes better, is actually preferred in Colombia.

Pork cooked in a microwave is particularly infective; because of uneven heating, microwaves don't always kill the trichinella. The United States Department of Agriculture recommends that pork cooked in a microwave reach a temperature of 170°F. This is particularly important for the internal parts of the meat.

BEEF

Raw beef is enjoyed in the form of steak tartare or carpaccio in some of the finest restaurants of the world; undercooked beef can produce beef tapeworm, a comparatively asymptomatic infection when compared to the harm created by the pork tapeworm. Rare steak and hamburger are risky as well. Undercooked beef or rare pork and lamb can also harbor toxoplasmosis. This disease is said to afflict the fast-food-eaters most of all because hamburgers are so often undercooked or prepared rare. The incriminating evidence can be hidden by mounds of ketchup, mustard, or mayonnaise. The wisest way to approach eating beef is to make sure your hamburger is well cooked with an internal temperature of 160°F. If you're eating a steak or roast, be sure the surface is also properly cooked.

FISH

The parasites most common to fish include fish tapeworms, anisakine larvae, and flukes. Freshwater varieties (mainly white fish) and a few inshore or migrating species like herring, mackerel, and salmon can be contaminated. In Finland, where raw smoked fish is popular, fish tapeworm is quite common, particularly from smoked salmon, causing a characteristic vitamin B_{12} deficiency, resulting in anemia and nervous-system disorders. Fresh Alaskan salmon is also commonly infected with fish tapeworm, which may be the reason there have been increased infection outbreaks noted in the western part of the United States. Cherry salmon, eaten by the more affluent in Japan for its delicious taste, has evidenced a similar fish tapeworm in that country. Besides salmon, other fish that carry tapeworm include pike, perch, lake trout, grayling, orange roughy, and turbot.

Anisakine larvae often reside in Pacific salmon, Pacific rockfish (red snapper), herring, and cod. When consumed raw (as in sushi, sashimi, and ceviche dishes), partially cooked, pickled, or smoked, these fish can transmit infection to humans. Salmon steaks as opposed to fillets are more likely to contain worms because they come from the abdominal area where more worms reside. Commercial blast-freezing seems to be the most effective way to kill larvae in fish, particularly in salmon and rockfish.

When anisakine larvae are ingested, they penetrate the walls of the stomach or small intestine, causing severe inflammation and pain. The symptoms can mimic appendicitis, gastric ulcer, or stomach cancer. Surgical removal of the worms is often required but can also necessitate removal of infected sections of the intestine. This type of surgery is common in Japan where raw fish is a dietary staple.

Of late, raw fish dishes—especially sushi and sashimi—have become more popular in the United States. In the *New England Journal of Medicine,* researchers have reported finding a new parasite that is transmitted to humans from fish. The eustrongylides worm had been thought to be found primarily in fish-eating birds. In the case reported in the journal, a 24-year-old student complaining of severe pain in his abdomen underwent surgery for appendicitis. The surgeons found a normal appendix. They also found a ten-inch pinkish-red worm, which crawled out onto the surgical sheets. The student was a once-a-month sushi and sashimi eater and most recently had eaten sushi at a friend's home. The majority of cases of eustrongylides worm have been reported from homemade sushi dishes, rather than from restaurant preparation.[8]

Because microwaves do not always cook evenly, fish cooked by this method are often underdone and can harbor live parasites. The *Journal of the American Medical Association* reported a case in 1988 of a woman who noticed some "thin, tan, paper-clip-length" worms squirming around in the uneaten piece of haddock she had cooked in her new microwave. Laboratory examination showed them to be anisakid worms.[9]

While this one woman may have changed her eating and/or cooking habits as a result of her experience, an entire nation revolted when they learned of the infestation of worms in native fish. In 1988, the West German fish market virtually collapsed overnight after a monthly public affairs TV program, *The Monitor,* aired an episode graphically showing closeups of worm larvae that had been removed from the bellies and flesh of fresh herring. Researchers said they had also found these live larvae in jars of pickled herring on supermarket shelves. The program director, who had aired the show in hopes the fish industry would improve its monitoring practices, was stunned that this one program could so radically change the eating habits of an entire nation.[10]

Liver and lung flukes are more common in Asia (China, Japan, Korea) because of the ethnic custom of eating raw or insufficiently cooked fish. Liver fluke comes from undercooked, salted, and dried raw fish. It has been found in carp, which is considered a delicacy among Orientals, as well as forty other species. Oriental lung flukes come from raw or inadequately cooked fish such as crabs and crayfish.

Other flukes, such as the intestinal fluke and sheep liver fluke can infect aquatic vegetation. Infections are common in China, Thailand, Vietnam, and India. The larvae of the intestinal fluke become encysted on water chestnut hulls, bamboo shoots, and lotus plant roots. The sheep liver fluke in its encysted larvae form attaches to water weeds and watercress, for example. Because these plants are often cultivated in ponds and streams, they can become infected by feces of neighboring cattle and sheep. Such cases have been reported in Latin America, the Middle East, and Australia.

CHICKEN

Among food-borne illnesses contracted from chicken, both salmonella and *Campylobacter jejuni* top the list. In fact, there are around 4 million campylobacter-related illnesses each year, making it the primary cause of bacterial maladies per the CDC. The symptoms typically include fever, diarrhea, and abdominal pain. And although these symptoms may disappear within five days, campylobacter illnesses have also been linked to a deadly nerve disease known as Guillain-Barré syndrome. The best line of defense is to be sure your chicken is well cooked to a 160°F internal temperature. (Chicken breasts should be cooked to 170°F internal temperature.)

STUFFING

It seems that every year around the holidays we hear of more cases related to salmonella contracted through stuffing. Since the bread drinks up the juices, it can become inundated with the bacteria and passed on to unsuspecting family members and guests. Diarrhea, cramping, and fever may appear within 12 hours or even up to three days afterward. Each year the CDC reports approximately 40,000 cases and 1,000 deaths from salmonella poisoning. Some of these cases clear up in about a week, but others may even require hospitalization. Be safe and cook your stuffed meat to 165°F internal temperature.

EGGS

Eggs pose yet another problem when it comes to salmonella poisoning. A particular strain called *Salmonella entiritidis* appeared between 1993 and 1994 in a nationally dispersed ice cream product. And in 1995 other products containing eggs were also found to have the strain. Stay on the side of caution and cook your eggs properly, making sure both the yolk and white are not runny. Using medium heat, scrambled or fried eggs should be cooked for at least two to three minutes.

BERRIES

Whatever the season here at home, we can now enjoy an array of fresh berries any time of the year, thanks to imports from foreign shores. That practice, however, has apparently increased our potential for parasitic infection. In 1996, 21 crates of raspberries from Guatemala were the source of a cyclospora invasion. And then, in 1997, strawberries imported from Mexico caused an outbreak of hepatitis A among teachers and children at a school in Michigan. Hepatitis A is a highly contagious virus that attacks the liver and produces fever, diarrhea, and jaundice. The key to protection is to make sure fruits and vegetables are properly washed. You may want to read the "Food Handling" section in Chapter 9 for specific details on how to cleanse your produce effectively and safely.

food preparation habits

It is not just the eating of food that causes problems. Food preparation habits need to be examined. Since most food-borne parasites arise from raw or undercooked animal foods, the first rule of thumb is to cook. The use of meat thermometers is recommended so that internal temperatures can be checked frequently. This is especially important in microwave cooking. When preparing a meat or fish dish, cooks should refrain from sampling the dish before it is thoroughly cooked. The frequent custom of sampling ethnic dishes (such as country sausage and gefilte fish) for seasonings during preparation can transmit trichinosis and fish worms into the human.

Cutting boards, especially wooden ones, and knives and forks that come into contact with raw, uncooked flesh food—i.e., red meat, fish, or lamb—should be disinfected after each item is prepared. The cutting board and silverware can cross-contaminate other foods such as fruits and vegetables. Dr. Hazel Parcells recommends that all utensils used in the preparation of foods (particularly of raw flesh) be cleansed with scalding water or a Clorox bath (see page 112 for a Clorox bath formula for all foods). Dr. Parcells suggests using a few drops of Clorox bleach in the final rinsing water for all kitchen utensils. Clorox bleach neutralizes the toxic effects of sprays, bacteria, viruses, and parasites, according to Parcells' research.

Even organic fruits and vegetables should be Cloroxed. Vegetables known to carry parasites include watercress, lettuce, and radishes, as well as leafy greens. Whether the food is organic or not, I instruct all my clients to give all food the Clorox treatment, to be 100 percent on the safe side.

While most people can understand that food and water are common pathways for disease transmission, the prospect that household pets can pass parasitic disease may come as a surprise to pet owners. The next chapter may very well be the most startling in the whole book.

5

man's best friend

Animals, just like humans, can become infected with parasites. Internally, contaminated water and food can spread the problem to our pets. Externally, animals become infected by parasites on their bodies, especially on their fur, because of exposure to infected animal wastes. Forgetting to wash your hands even one time after handling or cleaning up after your animal can transmit the parasite to you. Pets are a wonderful part of life. They provide comfort, companionship, protection, amusement, and unconditional love for their owners. Researchers suggest that people who own animals generally are healthier than those who do not.[1] Yet, pets, like humans, are often victims of serious infections that can unintentionally be passed on to their owners. In fact, there is a whole set of diseases classified as "zoonoses" (animal-transmitted diseases) in parasitology textbooks.

Diane Elliot, M.D., a researcher at the Oregon Health Science University in Portland, wrote in the *New England Journal of Medicine* that humans can become infected with at least 30 illnesses from their pets.[2] Phillip Goscienski, M.D., head of the Infectious Disease Branch of Pediatrics at the Naval Regional Medical Center, San Diego, reported to the California Medical Association that about 40 animal-transmitted diseases have been reported in this country and that infectious diseases transmitted by animals to man total 240. What he found remarkable was that these diseases are almost always unsuspected and unrecognized. He says, for example, that dogs transmit 65 known diseases; cats, 39; and horses 35. And while a physician would be likely to inquire about contact with animals with an ill zoo employee or experimental laboratory worker, the connection between a sick child and a new puppy is routinely missed.[3]

In 1977, the television program *60 Minutes* discussed children of the Appalachian Mountains who had been infected with a form of dog and cat roundworm that sometimes causes a disease called visceral larva migrans. It was only after the children had died and autopsies were performed that the cause of their swollen bellies, eye problems, and spleen and liver enlargements was found—dog worms.

Whatever the actual number of animal-transmitted diseases may be, the point is clear: Animals are major carriers of disease, and most physicians, let alone the general public, are unaware of this fact. Children, pregnant women, and those individuals with crippled immune systems may be the most adversely affected. In an article appearing in the *New York Post* on May 31, 1991, White House physician Dr. Burton Lee "voiced anger at those who say it is nonsense to talk about transmission of disease between people and their pets, pointing to his own experience as a clinician at Memorial Sloan-Kettering Cancer Center in New York. 'It is not nonsense,' he said, recalling a case where a family's dog got feline leukemia, two children later died of leukemia, and both parents got forms of cancer." New York pediatrician Dr. Stuart Copperman reports that in families where strep throat infection was persistent, the family pets, in 40 percent of the cases, were the carriers of the strep organism. Although the pets showed no symptoms themselves, when they were treated, the strep infections in the human family members cleared up.[4]

There are something like 110 million pet dogs and cats in this country. About half of all dogs may be infected with at least one or more parasites, including hookworm, roundworm, tapeworm, and heartworm. Considering these numbers, the potential for transmission of parasitic infection from animals to humans is high. All pups, for example, are born with the dog roundworm *Toxocara canis*. These roundworm eggs can be deposited in grass, playgrounds, parks, beaches, and sandboxes where toddlers can play and infect themselves by eating dirt or contaminated objects that may contain parasite eggs. Once swallowed, eggs can hatch larvae. While these larvae never mature to full-grown worms in the human host, they do travel to the liver and lungs as well as into the circulatory system, by way of which they can be passed to virtually any organ.

Dog and cat hookworm larvae can penetrate human skin, forming lesions on the skin at the point of entrance. This syndrome is known as cutaneous larva migrans. Feet, hands, buttocks, and the genital area are the most frequently involved areas. When the larvae die, in a month or two, the disease dissipates. Although not widespread, this disease is more prevalent in the South, where going barefoot makes contact with the larvae more likely.

In the soil, the eggs can become infectious within two weeks. Soil, grass, and shade help the eggs survive. They usually settle near the top of the soil in a silt layer, which protects them from destruction by sunlight. Toxocara eggs are very hardy and can survive for years, resisting the most perilous weather conditions of rain and snow. There are no chemicals that can kill all the toxocara eggs in soil. While contaminated soil is the primary direct source of infection, children can become infected from the coat of a puppy who has been playing in contaminated soil.

PERIL IN DOG DROPPINGS

Toxocara is a constant public health threat in the United States. Studies show that up to 20 percent of soil samples from parks, playgrounds, and schoolyards are contaminated.[5] Toxocara is one of the most common parasites of dogs and cats. It is a highly infectious parasite when you consider the enormous number of dogs and cats in this country. A single female worm can produce as many as 100,000 eggs per day. The environment can be contaminated with virtually millions of eggs since dogs, for example, can harbor several hundred roundworms per animal. All pups are born with roundworm—the most likely reason, by the way, for diarrhea, distended bellies, and lackluster coats. Both dogs and cats can continually become infected as the larvae are passed through the milk of the mother to the baby animal.

How many of us have brought home a young pup to grow up side by side with the kids? Young puppies from three weeks to three months of age create the greatest environmental hazard because they excrete large numbers of roundworm eggs. Most susceptible are children under the age of five, particularly those youngsters between 15 and 36 months.

In the vast majority of cases, there are no symptoms and dog roundworm infection in humans is self-limiting. I remember a case in which a two-and-a-half-year-old boy demonstrated symptoms of occasional wheezing, coughing, and bloating. A nutrition and health history revealed that the child had a habit of eating dirt and grass. A thorough exam by the child's pediatrician revealed a somewhat enlarged liver. Within three weeks, and without any specific treatment, except my recommendation that the child be supervised to control his dirt-and-grass-eating habit, the child completely recovered.

The disease caused by dog and cat roundworms is called visceral larva migrans and was first recognized in 1952. The disease is characterized by flu-like symptoms, continual abdominal pain, inability to gain weight, blood changes, cough, rash, and enlargement of the spleen and liver. The larvae can migrate through the lungs, muscles, brain, liver, and into the eye. In the more serious cases, tumors can appear in the eye, producing a condition called ocular larva migrans. This is actually a condition of trapped larvae in the retina of the eye. The symptoms include eye pain, strabismus (inability to focus simultaneously with both eyes), and loss of vision. This syndrome may be misdiagnosed as malignant retinoblastoma, resulting in the unnecessary removal of the eye.

Perhaps the best-known parasitic infection of all is the cat-transmitted disease toxoplasmosis, caused by *Toxoplasma gondii,* a very common protozoan parasite. Cats become infected with toxoplasma by eating mice, birds, or raw meat. Through their feces, they then pass the parasite, which can take up to two or three days to become infectious, to people. The oocysts (living eggs) can live up to four months in soil and up to eighteen months in water. Feces may contain potentially viable cysts for up to a year after their deposit. It is estimated that from 30 to 80 percent of domestic cats have the parasite but show no symptoms.

Toxoplasmosis usually produces few or no symptoms at all in healthy older children and adults. It can, however, clinically mimic other diseases such as mononucleosis and lymphatic disorders. Approximately half a billion humans have antibodies to *Toxoplasma gondii,* indicating they have been infected at one time or another with this parasite. Generally, the disease presents no problems except when it strikes a pregnant woman or an individual, like an AIDS victim or a person suffering from chronic fatigue and immune dysfunction syndrome (CFIDS), who has a compromised immune system.

When a woman becomes infected for the first time during pregnancy, especially in the first trimester, toxoplasmosis can pose a small but significant risk to the unborn baby. Stillbirths, miscarriage, and birth defects such as blindness, cleft palate, hearing loss, mental retardation, seizures, and cerebral palsy can result from congenital infection. Immunosuppressed individuals, particularly patients with AIDS, can develop fatal encephalitis from a toxoplasma infection. For these reasons, pregnant women and individuals with weakened immune systems should have somebody else empty the cat's litter box on a daily basis and should wear gloves when gardening.

Researchers at the federal Centers for Disease Control documented an outbreak of toxoplasmosis in 1977 at a riding stable in Atlanta. Of the 86 people who used the stable, 35 became infected. Doctors theorized that the disease was spread when stable dust, containing parasite eggs deposited there in cat excrement, was stirred up by the horses and breathed by the riders. Although all the victims recovered, one pregnant woman miscarried.[6] Toxoplasmosis is highly prevalent with over half the population in America infected but asymptomatic. As much as 90 percent of the population in Paris, France, carries the infection.[7] And although cats have been primarily blamed for the spread of toxoplasmosis, our culinary preferences for poorly cooked hamburgers and undercooked lamb and pork are much more likely the source of infection.

Humans are not the only animals who can pick up toxoplasmosis. Dogs can also become infected. They acquire the disease when they eat infected cat feces. Dogs, in fact, often become blind and neurologically impaired by this disease. Thus, it is important to make sure your dogs are not allowed to roam randomly. Keep as watchful an eye as you can on what goes into their mouths.

Other animal-transmitted diseases are connected to fleas. The fleas of both dogs and cats can spread tapeworm if unknowingly ingested by a human. A child's fondness for kissing a pet on the mouth or being licked by the pet creates a risk of swallowing egg-carrying fleas from the pet's mouth.

Swallowing infected fleas leads to intestinal infection. Rice-shaped particles that resemble pumpkin seeds in the human's stool may be a sign of dog
tapeworm, which can easily be mistaken for pinworms. It is important to
deflea household pets frequently.

Dog heartworm can be transmitted to humans by mosquitoes. While
fatal at times to dogs, dog heartworm is usually benign in humans. Heartworm is most often asymptomatic, although coughing may be a symptom.
After humans are bitten by infected mosquitoes, the worm usually remains
in subcutaneous tissue. Rarely do the larvae complete their life cycle. If
they do, they migrate to the lungs and produce a benign coin-like lesion. On
an X ray, this lesion may be misdiagnosed as lung cancer, leading to need-
less surgery.

Today both dogs and cats, like most other wild and domestic animals,
can also carry giardia. Puppies are especially prone to infection through
contact with contaminated water or infected animal waste. Unintentional
contact with dog feces can spread the disease to humans throughout the
household. Household pets and farm animals can also carry cryptosporidium, a diarrhea-causing protozoan, and contaminate humans.

keeping animals healthy

Taking on the responsibility of a pet is much like bringing up a child. These
animals are dependent on you for their well-being. You have to make sure
they eat properly; you have to clean up after them and transport them to the
vet. In fact, you have to decide if they are sick because, unlike a child, they
cannot tell you. Keep an eye out for the classic signs of infection: dull coat,
potbelly, poor growth, diarrhea, constipation, vomiting, fatigue, and anemia.
Since many parasitic infections in animals, like toxoplasmosis in cats, do
not produce recognizable symptoms at all, regular veterinary care is essential to maintain your pet's health.

Keeping your pets free of parasites and fleas is your best protection
against animal-transmitted diseases. Prevention is vital in the control of
roundworm infection because no chemical can yet kill all the toxocara eggs
in the soil. Like humans, healthy, well-fed animals can build up an immunity to many internal parasites. Being well-fed also makes animals such as

cats less likely to hunt and eat the animals that carry the *Toxoplasma gondii* organism, like mice and birds. Avoid feeding animals raw meat or raw fish, which harbor tapeworm.

Keep your pets vaccinated and have them periodically screened for parasites and fleas. Routine worming of pets is recommended. Worm at three months, then at six months, and then every six months thereafter. All worming medications contain dangerous compounds. Some pet owners have inadvertently killed their animals by worming them with over-the-counter medications. Don't be taken in by the advertisements for once-a-month, over-the-counter products. To evaluate and treat a parasitic condition in your pet properly, a licensed veterinarian is your best bet. The products recommended by the vet will vary depending upon the internal parasite diagnosed and the age and condition of the animal. Repeated treatment is often necessary because of the life cycle of the parasites. The initial deworming treatment is only effective against the mature adults and is not effective against the larvae or immature stages that are still in the animal's body at the time.

Simple commonsense measures can be taken to help prevent the risk of infection for you and your family. Be a "pooper scooper"; don't allow your animals to use the neighborhood as their bathroom; empty your cat's litter box daily; keep it and your animal's food and water dishes disinfected on a regular basis; buy flea collars or use topical insecticides.

Some individuals use pet manure in composting, not realizing the risks involved. Although I applaud the composting effort in general, there are hazards in using dog and cat feces in compost heaps. Composting cannot be relied on to remove the dangers from roundworm eggs. These eggs are very hardy and can contaminate dirt for years. Even after the fecal matter itself is no longer evident, the eggs will still be present. More complete information on preventive measures can be found in Chapter Nine.

It is possible to greatly reduce your risk of infection. If, however, preventive measures fail, you will need the information found in Chapter Six.

6

are parasites your problem?

Ultimately, each of us is responsible for his own health, and nowhere is this seen more dramatically than in the case of parasites. Parasitic infection remains a neglected disease. Physicians hardly ever suspect parasites as a current American health problem and, therefore, rarely ask for a comprehensive travel and lifestyle history. Without this kind of history, parasites—which can linger in your system for up to 30 years—can be easily missed because their symptoms mimic a host of diseases. As mentioned in Chapter One, irritable bowel syndrome and chronic fatigue may be cases of giardia. Persistent allergy is often a case of roundworm infection, while pinworms may be at the bottom of your child's hyperactivity. So a comprehensive personal history emphasizing travel and lifestyle habits is a vital link in determining the primary underlying cause of illness.

The questionnaire in this chapter is a lifestyle checklist designed to highlight the major avenues by which parasites are transmitted into the human body and to identify symptoms that commonly occur in parasite-based illness. This questionnaire can help you, along with your doctor, to assess your parasite risk. This basic questionnaire was first developed while I was working at an environmental detoxification center in San Diego, where parasitic screening was a standard part of total medical testing. Since so many patients were showing positive stool samples and couldn't understand why, the questionnaire helped them trace their sources of infection and pinpoint exactly how, when, and where they may have acquired parasites. Connecting the dates of symptom onset to a trip overseas or a new family pet can provide substantial clues for further health investigation.

Naturally, the more items you check off in this questionnaire, the greater the chances are that your health problems are parasite-connected. But remember, it may take only *one* exposure to tainted food, water, or the bite of an infected mosquito for infection to take place if your resistance is low.

Please answer the questions thoughtfully: "The life you save may be your own."

travel

○ Have you ever been to Mexico, Africa, Israel, China, Russia, Asia, Europe, or to Central or South America?

○ Have you traveled to Hawaii, the Caribbean, the Bahamas, or other tropical islands?

○ Do you frequently swim in freshwater lakes, streams, or ponds while abroad?

○ Did you serve overseas while in the military?

○ Were you a prisoner of war in World War II, Korea, or Vietnam?

○ Have you had intestinal problems, unexplained fever, night sweats, or an elevated white blood count during or since traveling abroad?

water

○ Is your water supply from a mountainous area?

○ Do you drink untested well water?

○ Have you ever drunk water from lakes, streams, or rivers on hiking or camping trips without first boiling or filtering it?

○ Do you use plain tap water to clean your contact lenses?

○ Do you use regular tap water that is unfiltered for colonics or enemas?

○ Can you trace the onset of symptoms (intermittent constipation and diarrhea, night sweats, muscle aches and pains, unexplained eye ulcers) to any of the above?

food

○ Do you regularly eat unpeeled raw fruits and raw vegetables in salads?

○ Do you frequently eat at sushi bars or salad bars; in delicatessens; vegetarian, Mexican, fish, Indian, Armenian, Greek, Pakistani, Ethiopian, Filipino, Korean, Japanese, Chinese, or Thai restaurants; fast-food restaurants; or steak houses?

○ Do you use a microwave oven for cooking (as opposed to reheating) pork, fish, or beef?

○ Do you prefer fish or meat that is undercooked, i.e., rare or medium rare?

○ Do you frequently eat hot dogs made from pork?

○ Do you eat smoked or pickled foods, e.g., sausage, lox, herring?

○ Do you enjoy raw fish dishes like sushi and sashimi, Latin American ceviche, or Dutch green herring?

○ Do you enjoy raw meat dishes like Italian carpaccio, steak tartare, or Middle Eastern kibbe?

○ At home, do you use the same cutting board for chicken, fish, and meat as you do for vegetables?

○ Do you prepare sushi or sashimi dishes at home?

○ Do you prepare gefilte fish at home?

○ Can you trace the onset of symptoms (weight loss, anemia, bloating, distended belly) to any of the above?

pets

○ Have you gotten a puppy recently?

○ Have you lived with, do you currently live with, or do you frequently handle pets?

○ Do you forget to wash your hands after petting or cleaning up after your animals, and before eating?

○ Does your pet sleep with you in your bed?

○ Do your pets eat from your plates?

○ Do you clean your cat's litter box?

○ Do you keep your pets in your yard where children play?

○ Can you trace the onset of your symptoms (abdominal pain, high white blood count, distended belly in children, unexplained fever) to any of the above?

workplace

○ Do you work in a hospital?

○ Do you work in a pet shop, zoo, experimental laboratory, or veterinary clinic?

○ Do you work with or around animals?

○ Do you work in a day-care center?

○ Do you garden or work in a yard to which cats and dogs have access?

○ Do you work in sanitation?

○ Can you trace the onset of symptoms (gastrointestinal disorders) to any of the above?

sexual practices

○ Do you engage in oral sex?

○ Do you practice anal intercourse without the use of a condom?

○ Have you had sexual relations with a foreign-born individual?

○ Can you trace the onset of symptoms (persistent reproductive organ problems) to any of the above?

major symptoms

Please note that although some or all of these major symptoms can occur in any adult, child, or infant with a parasite-based illness, these symptoms may instead be occurring as a result of one of many other illnesses.

ADULTS

○ Do you have a bluish cast around your lips?

○ Is your abdomen distended no matter what you eat?

○ Are there dark circles around or under the eyes?

○ Do you have a history of allergy?

○ Do you suffer from intermittent diarrhea and constipation, intermittent loose and hard stools, or chronic constipation?

○ Do you have persistent acne, anorexia, anemia, open ileocecal valve, skin eruptions, PMS, bad breath, itching, pale skin, chronic fatigue, food intolerances, sinus congestion, difficulty in breathing, edema, bloody stools, ringing of the ears, anal itching, puffy eyes, palpitations, vague abdominal discomfort, or vertigo?

○ Do you grind your teeth?

○ Are you experiencing weight loss or weight gain, loss of appetite, insomnia, depression, moodiness, sugar craving, lethargy, or disorientation?

CHILDREN

○ Does your child have dark circles under his eyes?

○ Is your child hyperactive?

○ Has your child been diagnosed with "failure to thrive"?

○ Does your child grind or clench his teeth at night?

○ Does your child constantly pick his nose or scratch his behind?

○ Does your child have a habit of eating dirt?

○ Does your child wet the bed?

○ Is your child often restless at night?

○ Does your child cry often or for no reason?

○ Does your child tear his hair out?

○ Does your child have a limp that orthopedic treatment has not helped?

○ Does your child have a brassy staccato-type cough?

○ Does your child have convulsions or an abnormal electroencephalogram (EEG)?

○ Does your child have recurring headaches?

○ Is your child unusually sensitive to light and prone to eyelid twitching, blinking frequently, or squinting?

○ Does your child have unusual tendencies to bleed in the gums, the rectum, or the nose?

INFANTS

○ Does your baby have severe intermittent colic?

○ Does your baby persistently bang his head against the crib?

○ Is your baby a chronic crier?

○ Does your baby show a blotchy rash around the perianal area?

If you answered "yes" to more than 40 items, you are at high risk for parasitic infection. If you answered "yes" to 30 items, your risk for parasitic infection is moderate. If you answered "yes" to 20 items, you are at risk. If you are not exhibiting any overt symptoms now, remember that many parasitic infections can be dormant and then spring to life when you least expect them. Be aware that symptoms that come and go may still point to an underlying parasitic infection because of reproductive cycles. The various developmental stages of parasites often produce a variety of metabolic toxins and mechanical irritations in several areas of the body—for example, pinworms can stimulate asthmatic attacks because of their movement into the upper respiratory tract.

typical case histories

While counseling the patients at the San Diego environmental detoxification center, I found that it was only after completing the questionnaire that most patients were able to trace the onset of symptoms to a trip to Mexico or overseas. Oftentimes, the patient was asymptomatic during the trip, then after being home for two to six weeks developed symptoms like massive bloating, gas, and intermittent diarrhea. Because of the delay in symptom development, the trip and symptoms had no connection in the patient's mind.

Had the patients been aware of travel-related parasite risks, they might have taken better precautions in the first place; or if symptoms did develop upon their return, they would have sought immediate medical attention, suspecting the most likely source of their problem. Because symptoms of parasitic infection are so similar to more familiar and recognizable diseases, making this connection reduces the chance of misdiagnosis.

With the inclusion of a purged stool sample from all incoming patients to screen for parasites, I discovered many were being treated for diseases they did not have. One gentleman, for instance, stated he was being treated for the past couple of years for peptic ulcer. After completing the question-naire, he realized his ulcer symptoms began shortly after a trip to China (where human feces are commonly used for fertilizer). A stool sample re-vealed this man had in his system a parasite called *Ascaris lumbricoides,* commonly known as roundworm, which often mimics peptic ulcer. The proper worm medication was prescribed, and the "peptic ulcer" soon disap-peared. There are many other problems roundworms can cause in the body that every individual should learn to recognize, such as bronchial symp-toms, abdominal pains, and intestinal blockages that can result in chronic constipation.

Another interesting case concerned a male patient whose allergy prob-lems became very severe after a trip to Mexico. Stool testing revealed this patient was infested with giardia, and soon after medication was given, his allergy problems decreased. Before treatment, this 35-year-old gentleman was allergic to almost 30 foods and had to curtail his exercise program and his work because of depression and severe fatigue. Within several days of taking the prescribed medication, he was eating foods he had not eaten in years and feeling like his old self again.

The patient was fine for three weeks, and then the phone calls to the clinic began again. Our client was beginning to suffer from his old prob-lems. Another stool sample revealed the presence of giardia cysts. Appar-ently the medication had not been strong enough to prevent the reproductive cycle, and the giardia had taken over his intestines once again. After another course of medicine, the patient was fine, and I believe he is still in good health.

unusual case histories

Some of the more unusual parasite-related cases I have heard of were shared with me by Dr. Abram Ber, a Phoenix, Arizona, homeopath. A small sampling of hundreds of his cases shows the enormous range of health problems that can be parasite-related.

Case number one concerns a two-and-a-half-year-old girl with a recurring fever of unknown origin and several months' duration. The child exhibited an elevated white blood count and a high SED rate, which shows tissue destruction. She had been taken to several pediatricians, and none could determine the cause of her symptoms. Finally, the mother came to see Dr. Ber. The child was still experiencing a 101°F to 102°F fever, was pale, and showed a poor appetite. When Dr. Ber took a comprehensive case history, he discovered that the child had a number of pets—seven cats and assorted chickens and rabbits—and habitually played naked with these animals. A rectal exam and lab tests revealed pinworms and toxoplasmosis. The child was treated with medication, homeopathy, and immune-boosting injections. Within 48 hours, her color and appetite improved, but the fever still persisted. Finally, after continued treatment under Dr. Ber's guidance, the fever subsided and the child recovered.

Case number two concerns a nine-year-old boy with severe behavioral problems and hyperactivity who was brought in to see Dr. Ber. After a complete examination that included testing for parasites, schistosomiasis was found both in the stool and the urine. Puzzled, Dr. Ber asked whether the child had been to Egypt (where schistosomiasis is the number-one health problem) or whether the child ate a lot of snails (freshwater snails are the parasite's intermediate host). The mother explained that the child played with snails from his backyard and was not in the habit of washing his hands before eating, despite her pleas. After the proper treatment was administered, the child's hyperactivity diminished and his behavior became normal.

Case number three concerns a woman in her late fifties suffering from such severe muscle pain that she was almost an invalid. Her medical history revealed that sixteen years prior she had lived with a family who ate a great deal of pork. During that time, she developed a flu-like illness accompanied by a high fever. Eventually, this illness went away, but severe aches and pains in the muscles remained. A blood smear showed trichinella, the pork worm that causes trichinosis, while the stool showed *Taenia solium,* or pork tapeworm. After she was treated for parasites, the woman became nearly pain-free.

As these case histories demonstrate, the importance of an in-depth personal history that examines both present and past travel, lifestyle, and dietary patterns cannot be overemphasized. Many diagnostic clues can be uncovered when the health-care practitioner asks the right questions and considers previous travel history in particular. The next chapter explains the newest and most advanced testing methods. Coupling those methods with the information derived from this questionnaire, a health-care practitioner can make a proper diagnosis.

7

diagnosis

The first step in diagnosing parasites is your physician's suspicion or your concern that parasites may be the root cause of your health problems. This requires a basic understanding of the geographic distribution, methods of transmission, symptomology, and life cycle of parasites. Clinical manifestations related to parasites include eosinophilia (an increase in the number of a certain kind of white blood cell), dysentery, diarrhea, itching, enlarged organs, anemia, and muscular aches and pains. A comprehensive travel, dietary, and lifestyle history is an essential diagnostic tool. The parasite questionnaire provided in Chapter Six can help you or your physician assess your parasite risk.

As far back as 1963, an article appeared in *Medical Tribune* entitled "Parasitic Disease Increases in U.S. from World Travelers Are Reported." In the article, Dr. Martin E. Gordon, a Yale investigator, demonstrates the importance of a physician's alertness to the geographic distribution and clinical manifestations of the common hookworm parasite. This awareness can aid in the early diagnosis of diseases of the modern traveler. Dr. Gordon gives the example of a Yale freshman with "vague abdominal cramps, occasional waves of nausea, and a striking picture of maternal dependence. . . . Knowledge of his eagle scout expedition to Africa the previous summer, when he lived with a pygmy tribe and walked barefooted, led to diagnostic stool examination. Hookworm therapy with dithiazanine rapidly cured his alleged psychoneurosis." Dr. Gordon suggests that the challenge is to promptly recognize the geographic prevalence of particular parasites and their symptoms so appropriate treatment can be initiated and complications avoided.

A strikingly dramatic example of the importance of physician alertness is the case of malaria. Reports of malaria here in the United States are on the rise, and strains are showing increasing resistance to the traditional drugs used for treatment. "In the United States, many of the deaths from malaria are the result of delayed diagnosis and treatment because the health care provider did not suspect malaria."[1] A thorough travel assessment should be done on any individual who has a fever and has within the last two years visited an area where the disease is endemic. Although most exposed individuals develop symptoms within six weeks, some may not manifest symptoms until a year after exposure, and relapses of malaria can occur up to two years after exposure.[2]

The traditional method for diagnosis of parasitic infection—the search for cysts, trophozoites, ova, eggs, or worm segments in a random stool sample—is inaccurate and misleading for several reasons. Parasites that reside in the tissue and blood, such as those causing malaria, filariasis, and trichinosis, will not be found in fecal samples. Parasites that are more prevalent in children, like pinworms and dogworms (visceral larva migrans), are also rarely seen in the stool. Pinworm eggs are generally not seen in the stool, and since dogworms are in the larval stage in a visceral larva migrans infection, there are no adults present to lay eggs that can be detected in the stool. To confound the situation further, many parasites do not appear in the stool because they dwell in the gastrointestinal tract lining (the lumen). These parasites strongly adhere to the intestinal mucosa. Unless they are somehow pulled out from the lining, they do not appear in stool samples.

In the case of some species—*Entamoeba histolytica*, giardia, and strongyloides, for example—cyst, egg, or segment excretion rate can vary from day to day. This is why most parasitologists suggest examination of three stool samples taken on different days. Parasite expert Dr. Louis Parrish even recommends that if these three samples are negative and clinical symptoms persist, three to six more samples should be taken.[3]

However, even when this practice is followed, the diagnosis can be missed. *Medical Microbiology* states:

> Unfortunately, a number of substances that may be administered to the patient in the course of diagnosis or therapy can impair the ability to make a direct diagnosis. These compounds can suppress the shedding of amebas into the stool but may not interfere with the course of invasive infection.
>
> Such compounds include barium, bismuth, kaolin, soapsuds enemas, and antimicrobials that reach the intestinal lumen. The suppression of shedding may be short-lived (soapsuds enema), or may last weeks or months (broad-spectrum antibiotics). *These compounds render direct diagnosis unreliable and often impossible.*[4]

But two groundbreaking findings are giving diagnosis of parasite infection a promising turn. The first exciting work is being done at Stanford University School of Medicine. Scientists there have been using computers not only to study the DNA of several parasitic species but to genetically fingerprint them. Their intent is to more easily define the type of infection an individual has, in an effort to better outline the mode of treatment required. Complementing that technology, scientists at Berkley are planning to manufacture what they call a "lab on a chip" that will contain these genetic fingerprints. Once achieved, physicians everywhere will have the data readily available for use on their office PCs.

The second important discovery is a stool antigen test. I've already shared with you how tricky it can be to detect the presence of *Entamoeba histolytica,* giardia, or cryptosporidium infections. Once these parasites stop shedding (after seven weeks in the case of *E. histolytica*), they can no longer be detected accurately. In fact, chronic cases sometimes produce a false negative stool exam. This new testing method is considered to be one of the most accurate methods available in determining pathogenic *Entamoeba histolytica,* giardia, and cryptosporidium infections. Using an immunofluorescent staining technique, this breakthrough method can detect the protein shell fragments of the actual parasite, normally not visible microscopically. It is, however, not an especially pleasant method of testing. So unless you're really determined, I would first suggest having a salivary GI test to determine the presence of *Entamoeba histolytica*. The salivary test (listed under the following Clinical Test section) may be particularly helpful during that non-shedding stage mentioned earlier.

Even with all these new findings, common sense would dictate that we use a variety of methods to confirm the suspected parasitic invaders present in the body.

clinical tests for parasites

Standing in the midst of this exponentially increasing epidemic, it is absolutely imperative that we all be properly tested for parasitic infection. However, there are differences of opinion on which method is the best mode of detection. The CDC currently recommends testing a minimum of three stool specimens as the most efficient means of detection—not using purged stool samples. Yet, it is not uncommon to find that some experts believe otherwise. To give you a better understanding of parasite detection, here are some of the more accurate modes of testing available today.

PURGED STOOL TEST

A purged stool test (used with a chemically induced stool as opposed to a random bowel movement) is probably the best all-around general method for identifying the majority of common parasites. This method of analysis is widely considered superior to normal random stool specimens, according to LuCrece Dowell, M. Sc.D., of Dowell Laboratories in Mesa, Arizona. Dowell perfected the method when she was a laboratory officer during World War II. She writes:

> If a patient had a feces examination during the initial or acute phase of dysentery (often amebic) the parasite was usually found and identified. The chronically ill patient with amebic hepatitis or amebic colitis was rarely diagnosable from a random stool examination. These cases were often suspected clinically but repeated random stool examinations failed to confirm the clinical opinion

and the patient was considered to have a simple spastic colitis, cause undetermined, or was unjustly judged a malingerer.

With the preceding problem in mind, a procedure utilizing extensive purging and extensive careful examination was worked out at an Army hospital, based on the invasive properties of one of the more pathogenic parasites, i.e., *Entamoeba histolytica*. Any type of colitis can be shown due to a pathogen when the stool examination is done on a specimen obtained by proper purging and examination allowing sufficient time.[5]

A purged stool test is particularly good for identifying the presence of giardia, amoeba, roundworm, threadworm, tapeworm, hookworm, cryptosporidium, liver flukes, blood flukes, strongyloides, and blastocystis. The procedure consists of taking 1.5 ounces of Fleet Phospho-Soda on an empty stomach to induce bowel movements. No red meat or red juice should be consumed for at least 24 hours prior to the purge. A light evening meal is suggested prior to the purge, and only clear tea or water should be drunk between that meal and the collection of the sample. Dowell found that parasites, regardless of their type, rarely appear before the fourth evacuation, and often as many as twelve bowel movements are required to yield a positive stool or to rule out parasite involvement. Generally, the labs testing purged stool samples will give instructions on which bowel movement to collect for the sample. After collection, the sample is placed in a container with a formaldehyde-based preservative for examination.

A purged stool is contraindicated in cases of gastrointestinal obstruction, pregnancy, appendicitis and debilitation. Since the saline laxative used for the purge is a high-sodium substance, individuals with high blood pressure must be careful. In this case, two to three tablespoons of Epsom salts in a large glass of warm water can be substituted for the Fleet Phospho-Soda.

BUENO-PARRISH TEST

The Bueno-Parrish method, originated by internationally renowned parasitologist Hermann R. Bueno, is a rectal mucus swab combined with specially developed immunofluorescent stains that identify giardia and cryptosporidium. This method is a good alternative for patients who prefer not to use a purged stool or have health problems that would be exacerbated by that method. Rectal mucus is obtained from the mucosa using a small rectal speculum. This simple procedure is easy to perform and has yielded a high positive rate even when the purged stool sample was negative.

A recent study shows that when this method of diagnosis was used, almost 50 percent of patients tested and previously diagnosed as having irritable bowel syndrome were, in reality, suffering from giardiasis. The patients tested had suffered with misdiagnosed bowel problems for an average of seven years.[6]

STRING TEST

If the purged stool and rectal mucus swab prove negative and giardia is still strongly suspected, other tests can be performed. These are the string test (Enterotest), duodenal aspiration, and duodenojejunal biopsy.

The most simple procedure, the string test, recovers a sample of duodenal fluid through the swallowing of a special gelatin capsule containing a string. One end of the string is secured to the patient's cheek while the other is attached to the capsule. After three to four hours, the string is withdrawn through the mouth and mucus is examined microscopically. This method can also be used to diagnose strongyloides.

BLOOD TESTS

Blood tests can be used to reveal an elevated eosinophil count, a general indicator for an infection by parasites—except for giardia and amoeba, which rarely cause eosinophilia. Roundworm, hookworm, toxocara, pinworms, and strongyloides often manifest a high eosinophil count. In fact, roundworm and hookworm can cause up to a 25 percent eosinophilia increase, whereas strongyloides may be the reason behind a greater-than-25-percent eosinophilia increase.[7] Many physicians dismiss elevated eosinophils as an indicator of allergy, not realizing the primary allergen is the parasite itself.

Abnormal levels of vitamins, minerals, and liver enzymes may indicate the presence of parasitic involvement. Low serum protein and potassium levels can indicate strongyloides; low levels of vitamin B_{12} may indicate fish tapeworm. Low folic acid, iron, and serum calcium may mean giardia, while low iron serum can signal the presence of hookworm. Alkaline phosphatase levels can be elevated in cases of amebiasis.

Blood tests are also used to determine malaria infection; microscopic examination will reveal parasitized red blood cells. Filaria can be diagnosed by identifying microfilariae in thick blood smears. These blood smears are best made at night, when levels of the organism are usually higher.

Available tests of the blood serum measure antibodies produced by the immune system in an attempt to fight off the parasite. These tests detect antibodies to organisms like *Entamoeba histolytica*; strongyloides; blood, liver, and lung flukes; toxocara; leishmania; *Toxoplasma gondii*; malaria; filaria; cysticerci; heartworm; and trichinella. Results of these antibody tests may not be entirely reliable with immunocompromised patients whose immune systems are so depressed that they cannot produce antibodies.

SALIVARY GI TEST

A salivary test is an excellent method for detecting *Entamoeba histolytica* and for determining mucosal immune response to certain proteins. These findings can be critical to the health of your gastrointestinal tract, since it can become inflamed due to allergic-type responses to certain foods and/or organisms. Among those antibodies tested are those for Gliadin (gluten protein), milk (mixed proteins), *Candida albicans, H. pylori* (the ulcer-causing bacteria), and Secretory IgA.

URINE TESTS

Urine testing can detect the presence of blood fluke eggs from urine sediment. Microfilariae in filarial infection can also be recovered from urine sediment. Examination of urine can frequently indicate the presence of *Tri-*

chomonas vaginalis in both females and males. In addition, urethral discharge can reveal trichomonas in men.

TISSUE SCRAPINGS AND SWABS

Perianal scrapings can be performed in cases of extraintestinal amoeba; material from the lesions is scraped and examined microscopically for evidence of the amoeba. Swabbing of the perianal area can be used to recover eggs of the pork tapeworm, beef tapeworm, and blood fluke.

The Scotch tape anal and perianal swab diagnosis is unique for the pinworm. Since the female adult worm lays her eggs around the perianal area in the early-morning hours, specimens are best obtained then, before you bathe or use the bathroom. Ordinary Scotch tape—or any other brand of transparent tape—is pressed against both sides of the anal and perianal areas and then transferred to a slide for microscopic examination.

RADIOLOGIC TESTS

A computerized axial tomography (CAT) scan or magnetic resonance imaging (MRI) of the brain can show brain lesions caused by toxoplasmosis and cysticercosis caused by porkworm. A CAT scan of the eye can show trapped larvae from ocular larva migrans, thereby disproving a mistaken diagnosis of retinoblastoma. A CAT scan of the liver can confirm amebic liver abscess. Common chest X rays can detect *Pneumocystis carinii* and dog heartworm, which appears as a coin-like lesion and has sometimes been mistaken for lung cancer. In many cases, ascaris can show up in X rays of the abdomen as outlines around intestinal gas pockets.

ASPIRATION

During aspiration, fluids are removed from a body cavity by suction. Rectal, liver, lung, and colon aspirations can reveal *Entamoeba histolytica*. Giardia and stronglyoides can be aspirated from the duodenum; giardia can also be aspirated from the gall bladder. Toxoplasma and leishmania can be aspirated from lymph node tissue.

BIOPSY

A biopsy is removal and examination, usually microscopic, of tissue from the living body. Muscle biopsy can reveal the larvae of both the trichinella and the cysticercus of pork tapeworm. Rectal biopsy can uncover flukes, while liver biopsy is used for visceral larva migrans. Needle biopsy can show heartworm lodged in the lung while lung biopsy detects *Pneumocystis carinii*. Lymph biopsy can uncover toxoplasmosis.

CULTURES

A culture is the propagation (breeding) of microorganisms or of living tissue cells in media conducive to their growth. Trichomonas can easily be cultured from vaginal samples. Worms in various life-cycle stages can also be cultured. Strongyloides are among the easiest parasites to culture from stool samples. Intestinal amoeba (such as *Entamoeba histolytica*) and Acanthamoeba can be cultured. Roundworm, blood fluke, and leishmania have also been successfully cultured through various life cycle stages.

PRENATAL TESTS

Prenatal diagnosis of toxoplasmosis can be accomplished by analysis of amniotic fluid and fetal blood as well as by ultrasound study (sonogram) of the fetal brain. This is a very important screening that can protect your unborn child from the devastating effects of congenital toxoplasmosis, which can cause mental retardation and blindness. All pregnant women should insist upon these tests.

In France and Austria, laws require that all pregnant women be tested for toxoplasmosis. Anti-toxoplasma antibodies can be examined with a new test, the Murex single use diagnostic system (SUDS). This test provides a very fast screening for outpatient settings and is of particular value for women before and during pregnancy. (During the yearly Pap smear, all women should insist upon screening for pinworms, ascaris, and filaria, which have all been found vaginally.)

DIAGNOSTIC TESTING

Diagnostic testing is performed by a variety of laboratories around the country and may also be done at home, using prepared kits. See the Resources section at the back of the book for contact information.

Uni Key Health Systems, Inc., is a distributor of a variety of products and services, including purged stool kits and/or salivary GI profile kits. Both come with complete step-by-step instructions. These tests can be performed in the privacy and comfort of your home. Uni Key also carries the stool antigen test kit. Uni Key has been my one-stop fulfillment center for books and products for my clients for more than seven years. I proudly promote their products because I have found them to be both gentle and effective. The certified parasite lab tests listed in the Resources section for over a dozen protozoans, fifteen types of worms, and common yeast culprits (such as *Candida albicans* and fungi spores). Another lab will test your salivary sample to determine the presence of *E. histolytica*. It will also test for other previously undetected food allergies and bacterial and fungal conditions to gauge immune response via the Secretory IgA of the mucosal lining.

treatment

Treatment for parasitic infection is not a "do-it-yourself" project. During treatment, many individuals experience detoxification symptoms on their road back to health. Nausea, gastrointestinal discomfort, and frequent trips to the bathroom are not uncommon. You want to be in good hands while going through this sometimes puzzling and uncomfortable process.

The question of whether to treat an asymptomatic carrier is often discussed in the medical literature. An asymptomatic carrier is an individual who is not exhibiting noticeable symptoms but is still a carrier of a parasitic infection, which could be passed on to others. Practically all researchers agree that the asymptomatic carrier should be treated because of the potential of infecting others. This is particularly important with infected children and food handlers. In some cases of parasite-based disease, the medication used to treat symptomatic individuals is not effective in the asymptomatic cyst carrier. Appropriate alternative drugs must then be utilized.

It is also believed that if one member of a family is infected, the entire family should be treated. People who live together can infect one another when making food for each other or sharing bathroom facilities. So it is a good idea to treat all household members as a matter of course.

general objectives of treatment

Treatment of parasitic infection must be geared to *eradicating* the parasites, rather than *relieving* the symptoms of infection. If the parasites are not eradicated, the infection will continue to cause untold damage to the system. Given a proper environment, a parasite colony can flourish to sometimes fatal proportions. And so there are some symptoms of infection that should be alleviated promptly to protect the host. Parasite-induced diarrhea from amoeba, cryptosporidium, or giardia needs to be treated immediately to prevent dehydration. In immunocompromised individuals (such as those with AIDS), diarrhea can lead to severe dehydration and even death.

There's one other vital concern I'd like to mention regarding eradicating *Cyptosporidium parvum*, which is a most persistent uninvited guest. Since this parasite invades the body on an intercellular level, infection is deeply embedded and may produce false negatives. Therefore, appropriate follow-up testing is critical. Experts suggest administering a stool antigen test three weeks after treatment. If this first test proves negative, another should be administered 60 days later. And if that test produces a negative, having a third follow-up test six months later is recommended. Then, having received three negatives thus far, one last stool antigen exam should be performed six months after the last to be completely certain the infection is gone.

treatment protocol

The best treatment protocol for the most commonly occurring intestinal parasites—roundworms, pinworms, and tapeworms—entails the following five steps, which should be carried out in conjunction with an experienced health-care practitioner who can guide you through the recovery process:

1. Cleansing the intestinal tract.
2. Modifying the diet.
3. Administering effective substances to eliminate the parasites.

4. Recolonizing the gastrointestinal tract with friendly bacteria.
5. Eliminating parasite risk factors from the lifestyle and environment to avoid reinfection.

Success in treatment is predicated on a number of factors. To begin with, the length of time the patient has been infected and his basic overall health are keys in determining the length of time necessary to achieve successful results. Oftentimes, repeated treatment is required for complete success, especially if the infection is of a long-standing nature. Patient cooperation, as with treatment for any illness, is crucial.

CLEANSING

It's not uncommon for the health of the gastrointestinal tract to be compromised by inflammation and irritants. Inflammatory reactions lead to increased permeability and malabsorption, which automatically posts a WELCOME sign for parasites. And because many parasites become embedded in the intestinal wall, no type of medication can effectively reach them until the mucus and encrusted matter lying over the worms are softened. So the first step in ridding the body of parasites is to cleanse the gastrointestinal tract naturally.

The intestinal cleansing process can be accomplished through the use of one or more of the following natural substances: rice bran fiber, alfalfa leaves, butternut root bark, fennel seed, licorice root, Irish moss, anise seed, peppermint leaves, cranberry, psyllium seed husk fiber, flaxseed fiber, apple or citrus pectin, and buckthorn bark. These substances act like a broom and sweep the debris out of the digestive tract. (Note: This cleansing would not be appropriate for the more exotic blood- and tissue-invasive parasites, which cause malaria, trichomoniasis, toxoplasmosis, schistosomiasis, filariasis, elephantiasis, and leishmaniasis.)

Without equal, psyllium seed husk fiber, flaxseed fiber, and bran fiber are gentle and effective bulking agents in the removal of accumulated wastes. Their extremely high water-absorbing capacity lubricates old fecal matter dried on the colon wall for a softer, more normal evacuation. And their tremendous swelling capacity lets them absorb toxins and waste materials stored in the body. Bulking agents must be taken with adequate amounts of water, so be sure to check the directions on the product label.

It's not unusual, once you begin the cleansing process, for the body to pass strings of mucus and worms from the colon. That's why the highly beneficial detoxifying fiber found in citrus pectin as well as naturally effective herbs is so important in absorbing toxins from the system. These herbs include cranberry powder (known for its anti-yeast properties); butternut root bark (one of the best and safest laxatives); fennel seed (to soothe the digestion and help against flatulence and heartburn); licorice root (a mild laxative/detoxifier to help heal the irritated mucous membranes of the intestinal tract); and peppermint leaves (to help relieve gas pain and aid digestion). And since we don't always eat the right foods, the third essential to attaining an effective cleansing system is to add a blend of enzymes to help promote the absorption and proper assimilation of nutrients, which is necessary to strengthen our resistance.

Although there are a variety of cleansing products on the market that may contain some of these ingredients, I highly recommend Super G.I. Cleanse. It's an advanced yet gentle formulation to eliminate toxins, promote regularity, increase energy levels, reduce gas and bloating, and increase nutrient absorption. This carefully blended product contains all the key herbs and important fiber I just mentioned, which are necessary to cleanse your system effectively. Super G.I. Cleanse also contains an enzyme blend to help with proper digestion, healthy flora essential for restoring nutrient absorption and proper elimination, and cranberry powder to help with pH balance—critical in protecting us from becoming a breeding ground for parasites, yeast, and other toxins that commonly affect our immune systems. (See Uni Key in the Resources section for ordering information.)

The Royal Flush

Colonic irrigation and home enemas can be a helpful adjunct in cleansing the colon. Colonic irrigation (sometimes called a high enema) is a procedure whereby a lukewarm water solution is irrigated into the entire length of the large intestine. The procedure, which dislodges and removes toxins over the entire length of the intestine, takes about 45 minutes and is usually performed in a professional office. Sanitary procedures and ingredients, such as filtered water and disposable specula, are essential.

For those who prefer the do-it-yourself method, home enemas can be effective. Remember, however, that enemas reach only the lower 12½ inches of the 5½-foot colon, whereas colonic irrigation cleanses the entire length of the colon, up to the ileocecal valve.

Numerous home remedies can be added to enemas to make them more effective. Garlic's well-documented anti-parasitic properties make garlic juice enemas a beneficial treatment in cases of pinworms in children and adults. Garlic's active component, allicin, seems to be the substance that has the anti-parasitic properties.[1]

The Reverend Hanna Kroeger, a well-respected herbalist from Boulder, Colorado, suggests an enema of two mashed garlic cloves boiled in six ounces of milk and given for three consecutive nights to kill pinworms in children. Garlic enemas are also good because they support the normal acidity of the colon. Vinegar enemas (two tablespoons of apple-cider vinegar to one quart of water) are also helpful as general detoxifiers. Blackstrap molasses enemas (one tablespoon to a quart of water) will actually pull encrusted fecal matter and some parasites off the intestinal wall. Coffee enemas, used in detoxification programs, are helpful in cleansing the liver but can cause tissue weakness with prolonged use.

A word of caution when taking enemas: Use only properly filtered water, or purchase distilled water and further sterilize it by heating to a rolling boil for at least ten minutes. Sterilize the tubing and enema bag by soaking them in a diluted Clorox bath (half a teaspoon of Clorox for each gallon of water) for fifteen minutes. Rinse thoroughly with sterilized water. This procedure prevents the further introduction of water-borne parasites into your body.

Most general cleansing programs advocate the reintroduction of beneficial bacteria into the intestinal system. However, when cleansing for parasites, the protocol changes. In cases of giardia, for example, the parasites often cover complete parts of the small intestine, mechanically overcoming the normal bacteria flora. According to Great Smokies Diagnostic Laboratory, optimum bowel flora function is accomplished by destroying any parasites and pathogens.[2] So it is advisable to replenish beneficial flora after the microorganism is eradicated. Recolonizing the bowel with friendly flora is a final step, taken only after the medications used have been clinically proven successful in eradicating the problems (see page 105).

MODIFYING YOUR DIET

To date, there has been very little research regarding nutrition and parasitic-based disease in humans. Results of studies on nutritional interactions during human parasitic infections give us conflicting data. Simply put, better nutritional status helps the parasite's existence *and* improves the host's defense system. Poor nutrition will starve the parasite but will also weaken the host's immunity. There is limited definitive information for specific nutritional recommendations. Complicating variables—such as single infections being rarely observed, different parasite species affecting nutritional status in similar ways, individual parasitic organisms optimizing their own survival in several different ways while modifying their host's nutritional status, and cultural/socioeconomic variables—make definitive conclusions difficult.[3]

There are studies that have shown interference with vitamin A absorption when roundworm or giardia is present. This absorption problem is normalized after elimination of the worms, with or without supplementation with vitamin A.[4,5] In addition, during hookworm infestation, the severity of iron deficiency anemia has been shown to be proportionate to the number of worms present. The more severe the infestation, the more severe the deficiency. After elimination of hookworms, you should follow a high-protein diet with a daily supplementation of 50 to 100 milligrams of ferrous sulfate (taken after meals) for a minimum of three months or until hemoglobin levels return to normal.[6]

Fish tapeworms compete for vitamin B_{12} in the host. After the tapeworms are eliminated from the body, it can take up to one year for B_{12} levels to return to normal.[7] It is therefore important that you are patient in replenishing body supplies and are consistent in a day-to-day rebuilding of reserves. You may have been carrying around this uninvited guest for several years, so it will take some time to regenerate your system.

Despite the lack of definitive clinical human studies regarding the role of nutritional status in preventing or combatting parasite-based diseases, basic common sense and professional experience dictate certain sound nutritional practices. In my opinion, the cleansing program should be accompanied by a therapeutic diet that supports the host and starves the parasite. Diet strongly influences the intestinal environment. A diet high in simple carbohydrates like sugar, white flour, and processed foods can provide the ideal feeding ground for worms. Even so-called "natural sweets"—honey, barley malt, fruit, fruit juice sweeteners and concentrates—taken in excess can provide instant food for your internal hitchhikers. Fiber-deficient foods may have initially precipitated a breeding ground for parasites. These foods require more time to pass through the alimentary system. A sluggish transit time allows more food to decay and putrefy, thus producing stagnation in the colon and an inviting environment for parasites.

A Supportive Therapeutic Diet

In my fifteen years of experience with clients, I have found that a diet composed of 25 percent fat, 25 percent protein, and 50 percent complex carbohydrates works well for parasite-ridden bodies. The diet must have sufficient unprocessed oils (at least one to two tablespoons daily) from 100-percent expeller pressed safflower, sesame, flax, and canola oils. These oils lubricate the gastrointestinal tract and serve as a carrier for fat-soluble vitamin A. It appears that of all vitamins and minerals, vitamin A best increases resistance to tissue penetration by parasite larvae.[8] Animals fed diets deficient in vitamin A have shown an increase in tissue penetration by parasitic larvae.[9,10] Foods rich in vitamin A, such as cooked carrot, squash, sweet potatoes, yams, and greens, should therefore be amply included in the diet.

Eating sufficient, properly cooked protein (meat, fish, chicken, eggs) is vital to a supportive therapeutic diet. Protein provides the amino-acid building blocks necessary to strengthen tissues and enhance immunity. Studies show that children who suffer from malnutrition caused by roundworms benefit from increased protein intake.[11] Thus, a moderately-high-protein diet of well-cooked turkey, chicken, fish, and lamb that is easily digested, with lots of cooked vegetables, stews, and soups, may be the best therapeutic diet. For vegetarians, Multiminophan, a multiple source of natural free-form essential amino acids, can be used as a protein supplement. Mul-timinophan is available from Uni Key Health Systems (see Resources section).

Vegetarians and others who depend upon protein sources such as beans, nuts, seeds, peas, and legumes will need to restrict their intake of such foods. These high-fiber foods, in the presence of parasitic infections, cause flatulence and irritate the gastrointestinal tract. This further prevents the absorption of nutrients. However, because research has shown that a high-fiber diet helps prevent giardiasis,[12] a water-soluble fiber supplement that is gentler to the gastrointestinal tract is recommended. Less irritating fiber supplements include psyllium seed husks, rice bran, and oat bran.

Soy products such as tofu and tempeh can be included in moderation, i.e., not more than once or twice a week. Soy products leave an alkaline residue in the system, and it has been my experience that in parasite diet therapy, the system needs to be more acidic on a cellular level. An overly alkaline condition in the gastrointestinal tract provides a favorable environment for protozoans and worms.[13] Because several parasites, like round-worm and giardia, precipitate secondary lactose intolerances that sometimes persist after elimination of the parasites, limiting or completely avoiding dairy products during and after treatment may be necessary. Because of the damaged intestinal villi, giardia can also produce gluten intolerance—the inability to digest the protein portion of wheat and rye and, to a lesser degree, oats and barley. With any protozoan infection that can damage the intestinal villi, it is always a good idea to reduce the intake of grains (with the exception of gluten-free rice and millet).

Heavy intake of raw fruits and vegetables should be greatly curtailed, and cold or iced foods and drinks should be avoided. These foods cause the intestines to contract, thereby holding in toxins rather than releasing them. For the therapeutic parasite control diet, cook most fruits and vegetables so they will be more easily digested and more soothing to the intestinal tract. Raw vegetable and fruit juices are not suggested at this time.

A well-balanced, supportive eating program is essential because malab-sorption often occurs from parasitic damage to the intestine. Especially common in parasite infections is decreased absorption of fats and proteins and decreased absorption of vitamins, including beta-carotene, vitamin A, folic acid, and vitamin B_{12}.[14] A graphic example of this nutritional interaction between host and parasite can be seen in the case of the fish tapeworm. The adult tapeworm is "able to obtain as much as 75 to 100 percent of the physiological dose of vitamin B_{12} before the vitamin is absorbed by the mucosa."[15]

Eating the right foods, however, may not be enough to ensure proper nutritional support. Many people lack an adequate supply of the digestive enzymes that are needed to release the nutrients contained in foods. Even with a good diet, enzyme deficiencies can lead to nutritional deficiencies and weakened resistance.

Enzyme deficiencies also lead to incompletely digested foods that can putrefy or ferment in the intestines, creating an environment that is ripe for parasites. Concentrated plant enzymes from aspergillus (a fungal-type microorganism used in the fermentation of miso and soy sauce) can be used as a dietary supplement to help correct the underlying conditions that favor parasitic infections.

ADMINISTERING ANTI-PARASITIC SUBSTANCES

Besides the basic diet recommendations, there are special foods that have time-tested anti-parasitic properties. Among these are fresh pineapple and papaya, which contain high amounts of natural protein-digesting enzymes like bromelain and papain and have long been used by natives of Mexico to cure worm infestations. Because of the sugar content of these fruits, it may be better to take them in supplement form in which the extracts are often combined with pepsin and hydrochloric acid, which aid not only in food digestion but in digestion of the parasites. In cases of giardia, digestive enzyme supplements containing ox bile or bile salts should be avoided, as recent research reports that bile sparks the growth of giardia and bile salt is eagerly devoured by the parasite.[16]

Pomegranate juice, up to four glasses per day, available in health food stores or made at home with your juicer, is effective against tapeworm infection. In Mexico, papaya seeds are used for their parasite-eliminating powers. Fresh or dried, you may take a tablespoon daily (on an empty stomach) for one week. Then wait two days and repeat the amount for another week. They are also great to add in salad dressings, since their peppery taste adds a little zip. Eating a handful of pumpkin seeds or a porridge made from ¼ to ½ cup finely ground pumpkin seeds daily for four to six weeks can help eliminate a variety of worms. In fact, Native Americans often chewed pumpkin seeds as an effective deworming agent (vermifuge). Garlic has been used since ancient times as a vermifuge. Two cloves of raw garlic per day used in food preparation can be effective against roundworms, pinworms, tapeworms, and hookworms in both humans and animals. Onions, carrot tops, radish roots, kelp, raw cabbage, ground almonds, blackberries, pumpkin, sauerkraut, and fig extract also have anti-parasitic qualities.

In addition, lemon seeds (crushed) can be taken for five straight days as a parasite-fighting agent. You'll need to wait two weeks after the first five-day use, then repeat the process. Certain teas are also helpful in combating parasitic invasion. Try two to three cups of mugwort tea daily for two weeks. Or try this Asian favorite: three-taste tea, made from shakosai, licorice, and daio. Drink it three times daily for one week, one half hour before meals. Then wait two weeks and repeat the process. One other tea you may want to use is Corsican seaweed tea. Drink one cup daily for ten days, then wait two weeks and repeat the process.

Herbal Cures
Many effective herbs have been used by both eastern and western cultures to kill and expel parasites and worms. Some of the most effective include elecampane root, garlic, black walnut bark (including the kernel and green hull), butternut root bark, alfalfa leaves, licorice root, Irish moss, anise seed, peppermint leaves, buckthorn bark, pink root, goldenseal, wormwood, sage, cloves, tansy, fennel, thyme, cranberry powder, oil of oregano, and male fern. Some of these herbs, like fennel, thyme, sage, and garlic, can be used for seasonings in everyday cooking. Others are commonly available at health food stores in capsules, powders, and tinctures. Directions for use can be found on product bottles. Most herbal formulas on the market are usually taken before meals (presumably to immobilize the parasite before food is ingested) and sometimes before bedtime for ten days to two weeks.

Folklore instructions suggest that any course of treatment for worms should begin around the full moon, when the parasites supposedly become more active in the system. When beginning herbal treatments, it is a good idea to start with low doses for a few days to assure that there are no individual sensitivities. After the full course of treatment, allow the body to cleanse itself naturally before attacking the next reproductive cycle of internal boarders with another course of herbs.

Over the years, I have researched, experimented with, and written about various products. My clients and readers have reported very satisfactory results with several natural preparations. All the preparations mentioned in the following paragraphs can be ordered from Uni Key Health Systems. (See the Resources section.) Two such products developed by Uni Key, Verma-Key, and Verma-Plus are both effective against worms and flukes. Verma-Key, which is in capsule form, contains black walnut, wormwood, balmony, wormseed, cascara sagrada (a laxative), slippery elm, garlic, and cloves. Verma-Plus is a liquid herbal tincture containing black walnut, wormwood, centaury, male fern, orange peel, cloves, and butternut in a base of 20-percent alcohol and water. In most cases these two formulas work well together. It is recommended to take 2 to 4 Verma-Key capsules 20 minutes before meals 2 to 3 times daily with at least an 8-ounce glass of water followed by taking 5 to 20 drops of Verma-Plus in 2 ounces of water 2 times daily between meals and one time before bed. This program should be followed for two weeks. After two weeks there should be a 5-to-12-day rest period. Then repeat again for an overall total of 2 to 4 two-week intervals. In most cases this seems to be a sufficient time of treatment, although each person's situation may be different.

Two other such products designed by Uni Key for microscopic parasites (protozoa) are Para-Key and Para-Plus. Para-Key, which is in capsule form, contains cranberry concentrate, grapefruit seed extract, artemesia annua, garlic, cayenne, slippery elm, and bromelain. Para-Plus is a liquid herbal tincture containing black walnut, artemesia annua, prickly ash bark, quassia bark, cloves, and cranberry concentrate in a base of 20-percent alcohol and water. In most cases, these two formulas work well together. It is recommended to take 2 to 4 capsules of Para-Key 20 minutes before meals 2 to 3 times daily with at least 8 ounces of water followed by taking 5 to 20 drops of Para-Plus in 2 ounces of water 2 times daily between meals and one time before bed. This program should be followed for 2 weeks. After this time there should be a 5-to-12-day rest period. Then repeat again for an overall total of 2 to 4 two-week intervals.

In general, this treatment works well for most microscopic parasites. However, for stubborn cases of *Blastocystos hominus* I also recommend an additional supplement known as Undecylenic acid (derived from castor bean oil). This supplement comes in the form of capsules which should be taken right before each meal.

Homeopathic Remedies

There are also several homeopathic remedies for parasitic infections. Homeopathy, a healing process that has been practiced in Europe for almost 200 years, is based upon the premise that "like cures like." Homeopaths believe that any substance capable of inducing symptoms in a healthy individual will, in minute amounts, remove those same symptoms in a diseased person. Among homeopathic remedies for parasite infection are the following:

Remedy	Parasite or condition
Chelidonium	liver flukes
Chenopodium	hookworm / roundworm
Cina	pinworm
Felix mas	tapeworm
Santoninum	roundworm / threadworm

Other homeopathic remedies that are anti-parasitic include the tissue-cell salts sodium phosphate and calcium phosphate. The cell salt natrum sulphate is a well-respected systemic tonic for parasitic conditions.

As a temporary treatment for nausea resulting from amoeba and giardia infection, the homeopathic 6x potency of ipecacuanha can be used. While the full-strength ipecac syrup is used to induce vomiting, the homeopathic dilution causes no adverse reaction and is quite successful in alleviating nausea. It is best that homeopathic remedies be selected and used under the guidance of a qualified homeopathic physician or naturopath.

Effective Drugs

Many effective drugs are used against parasitic infections. In the appendix, I have included a protocol for physician reference from *The Medical Letter on Drugs and Therapeutics*. As the *Medical Letter* states:

> In every case, the need for treatment must be weighed against the toxicity of the drug. A decision to withhold therapy may often be correct, particularly when the drugs can cause severe adverse effects.[17]

The *Medical Letter* includes a very comprehensive listing of the adverse effects of some anti-parasitic drugs. Metronidazole (Flagyl), for example, used in the treatment of giardiasis, amebiasis, and trichomoniasis, can cause nausea, headaches, disorientation, and a metallic taste in the mouth. In addition, Flagyl encourages yeast growth, thereby wreaking more havoc on an already compromised immune system. Parasite expert Dr. Louis Parrish writes in the *Townsend Newsletter* with regard to parasites that many physicians are under the misconception that

> . . . treatment with a single course of metronidazole (Flagyl) is 90% effective. The facts: 25 years ago this may have been true, but the protozoa rapidly become resistant. Today the single course cure rate is less than 5%. Furthermore, approximately half of the patients treated with metronidazole complain of side effects, and 10% flatly refuse to take it ever again.[18]

In light of this, some physicians are choosing to use more natural remedies that have proven to be safer and just as effective. Patients report good success with these remedies and minimal side effects.

RECOLONIZATION OF THE INTESTINAL TRACT

Reintroduction of friendly bacteria in the intestinal tract following the complete eradication of foreign visitors is the final step in natural treatment methods. These friendly flora help detoxify noxious substances, maintain proper pH, and act as natural antibiotics against infectious bacteria. Thus, along with continuation of proper diet and lifestyle habits, can protect the body against future invasions.

The bacteria strains I have found most helpful in recolonizing the bowel include *Lactobacillus acidophilus, Lactobacillus bulgaris, Lactobacillus bifidus,* and *Streptococcus faeceum.* Many people need one or a combination of all four to repopulate the intestinal tract. There are many high-quality, hypoallergenic acidophilus-type formulations on the market. My patients have reported good results using Aqua Phase, a homeopathic anti-yeast liquid formula that reduces yeast overgrowth and allows beneficial bacteria to regenerate. Aqua Phase is available through Uni Key Health Systems. (See Resources section.)

A new breakthrough product for the recolonization of the intestinal tract is now available in the United States. The product is known as Dr. Ohhira's Probiotics 12 Plus and is named after Dr. Iichiroh Ohhira, a renowned microbiologist in Japan. His probiotic product is the most unique probiotic product in the world today. Probiotics 12 Plus contains a proprietary blend of 12 unique strains of live lactic acid bacteria that maintain the optimum pH in the colon to combat pathogenic bacteria like *E. coli.* Plus, this completely nondairy and organic product is the *only* probiotic I have found that also provides a special strain of lactic acid bacteria that has been proven in vitro to kill the most virulent antibiotic resistant superbugs like *Staphlococcus aureus.* The best news of all for worldwide travelers like me is that the product has a shelf life of more than five years and does not require refrigeration due to the unique encapsulation process that Ohhira developed.

Based upon just some of the clinical studies I perused as well as the testimonials I reviewed, Dr. Ohhira's Probiotics 12 Plus has been shown to stop diarrhea in its tracks, smooth out spastic colon attacks, decrease bloating and heartburn, inhibit yeast, improve sleep, boost energy, assist liver function, and support healthy digestive function. It appears to be ideal for traveling and the assurance of continued good health. I was so impressed with Dr. Ohhira's products that I agreed to become a spokesperson for the company.

When I first discovered the product, I started out with five capsules twice a day for a week. I am now on a maintenance dosage of two capsules twice a day. When I travel, however, I go back to the five capsules twice a day, just in case. This is the exact protocol I suggest for all my clients. (See Resources section.)

ELIMINATION OF PARASITE RISK FACTORS

This part of the treatment program is truly do-it-yourself because I have no straightforward answers. Only you can uncover the reason(s) you played host to parasites in the first place. Take a look back at Chapter Six and review the questionnaire once again. Do you frequently travel to exotic foreign locales and live like the natives? Are you a sushi lover? Do you like your meat extra rare? Are you in the habit of kissing your dog? Does your water come from a natural mountain spring?

Take responsibility for changing lifestyle, food, and environmental habits that put you in harm's way. The next chapter offers very specific guidelines to assist you in this process.

9

prevention

This is the most important chapter in the book. Since parasites are difficult to find, and often more difficult to treat, the best solution is to prevent them in the first place. Since some of them, like giardia, are fast becoming a fact of life, we will have to learn to live with them by strengthening our resistance to them. Parasites are opportunistic critters. Any flaw or weakness in our defense systems is an open invitation to invasion.

Our best line of defense against parasitic infection is a strong, healthy immune system. But our immune systems have taken a beating in the past few decades. Every year, 2.6 billion pounds of pesticides are used in the United States, mostly on food crops. The food we eat, instead of nourishing our bodies, challenges our immune systems with residues from these pesticides. Unless we take the time and care involved to clean our fresh fruits and vegetables as outlined later in this chapter, these very healthful foods can be the vehicle by which parasites enter our bodies, along with chemical and pesticide residues.

The groundwater supplies in over half the states in this country have been contaminated with pesticides from runoff. And, as discussed in Chapter Four, many municipal water supplies are antiquated and have become breeding grounds of giardia, bacteria, viruses, lead, and other contaminants. Even the air we breathe contains pollutants that challenge our immune systems. Each challenge to the immune system stimulates it into action. Parasites, as foreign invaders, also activate the immune response. As the parasites continue their invasion unchecked, the damage they cause to the body's vital systems, including the gastrointestinal and nervous systems, creates further stress on an already weakened immune system. This continual assault and damage eventually leads to immune system exhaustion.

Supporting our immune systems with foods rich in vitamins C, E, and beta-carotene and the minerals zinc and selenium is a good first line of defense against parasitic infection. Additional supplementation with these vitamins and minerals and with herbs like echinacea, ginseng, and astragalus is good insurance for a healthy immune system. These vitamins, minerals, and herbs have been shown in numerous studies to enhance and support immunity.

Since most parasites enter the body orally, one of the body's best defenses against them is our stomach acid. Very few pathogenic microorganisms can survive the hydrochloric acid in a healthy stomach. However, numerous factors lead to a lack of hydrochloric acid in the body:

- An overgrowth of *Candida albicans* can damage the cells that produce hydrochloric acid. A course of antibiotics can often result in an overgrowth of *Candida albicans,* leaving one of our body's best defenses against parasites severely weakened.
- Recent research has shown that people with type A blood have a genetic predisposition to a condition known as achlorhydria, whereby the body does not produce enough hydrochloric acid.
- Lead, one of the more toxic heavy metals widely distributed in our environment, binds the hydrochloric acid in our stomachs, making it unavailable for digestion.

Like the prevention of other major health problems, the prevention of parasitic infections must begin with the awareness that we are all at risk, even if we never travel outside the United States. By following the guidelines in this chapter in regard to personal and household hygiene, travel, sexual practices, food and water, day-care and school sanitation, household pets, and eating out, you can protect yourself and your family. I have put these guidelines into an outline form for easy reading and reference. At first they may seem overwhelming to some people. But the good news is that many of the common avenues of transmission are within our control. Armed with the proper information and education regarding our current-day environment, hygiene, sanitation, and food, we *can* overcome.

personal hygiene

We often overlook the importance of personal hygiene. Here's a reminder.

- *Always* wash your hands prior to eating.
- Make sure to wash your hands with soap and water after going to the bathroom, changing the baby's diaper, or handling your pets.
- Be sure to keep fingernails short and scrub under them. (A nail brush kept in the bathroom is a good idea.)
- Don't sit on a bare toilet seat without first wiping it or protecting it with toilet paper. Better still, squat. Pinworm eggs and trichomonas can lurk under toilet seats. Trichomonas can also be spread through mud baths, water baths, and sauna benches.
- Don't use tap water to clean contact lenses. Distilled water can also be contaminated, so buy sterilized lens preparations for all cleansing and disinfecting purposes. Make sure to remove contact lenses before swimming.
- Don't walk barefoot, especially in warm, moist, sandy soil.
- If you travel frequently, eat out on a regular basis, have pets, or live in a mountainous region of the country, have a complete parasite examination at least twice a year. The most accurate diagnosis comes from a combination of purged stool and rectal mucous exam. (See Chapter Seven.)

infant and child care

Healthful habits should be practiced and taught at the earliest stages of childhood.

8dd

Stopಸ

- Breast-feed your baby as long as you can. Human milk has anti-protozoan properties, which provide antibodies that fight against amoeba and giardia.
- Keep toddlers away from puppies and kittens that have not been regularly dewormed.
- Be sure your child routinely washes after contact with household pets. With infants, the task is *your* responsibility.
- It's a good idea to prevent toddlers from kissing household pets or being licked by them.
- Do not allow children to eat dirt.
- Do not allow children to play in yards, playgrounds, or sandboxes in which animals are allowed to roam loose.
- Clean children's bedrooms with a damp mop or vacuum to avoid stirring up possibly infested dust.
- Sanitize all toilet seats and bowls, but particularly those used by children, with a mild Clorox solution. Clean the undersurface of the seat.
- Clean children's toys with mild, soapy water.
- Keep children's fingernails short and clean.

PROCEDURES FOR AN INFECTED CHILD

Children who have pinworms should follow these additional preventive measures to avoid the spread and reinfection among other family members. These tips come from Leo Litter, M.D., a pediatrician in West Hartford, Connecticut:

- Bathe daily.
- Use one washcloth and towel for the face and hands, another for baths.
- Scrub hands thoroughly after bathroom use and before each meal.
- Wear close-fitting underpants at all times (under sleeping garments too).
- Do not share a bed.

PROCEDURES FOR AN INFECTED CHILD'S CAREGIVERS

Mom and Dad can help by instituting these additional measures:

- Launder bedclothing and personal clothing of the infected person daily.
- Keep toothbrushes in containers (thus avoiding exposure to bathroom dust that transmits pinworms).
- Scrub toilet seats daily.
- Clean and vacuum daily (to remove eggs along with the dirt).
- Keep all rooms—bedrooms, especially—well aired.
- As frequently as practical, superheat the home to 95°F for a day. Dr. Litter suggests this is the most effective way to kill embryos in the eggs. He suggests the children's rooms be heated to 95°F for just a day, preferably on a weekend when the family members are out.

water usage

Avoid water-borne disease by paying careful attention to what you drink.

- Check the status of your local water system. Violation and enforcement data on specific systems can be learned via the EPA's Web site: www.epa.gov/OGWDW/dwinfo.htm. You may also want to contact your local water supplier or state agency.
- Have your tap water tested. The EPA Safe Drinking Water Hotline can tell you who to contact. In Alaska and Washington, D.C., call (202) 382-5533; elsewhere, call 1-800-426-4791 between 8:30 A.M. and 4:30 P.M. EST.
- Drink only filtered water. It takes a fine-pore filter of not more than three microns to filter microorganism cysts. In a study conducted at Colorado State University in Fort Collins, Colorado, Royal Doulton (model F303) was among the four filters found to block giardia cysts from tap water. Through a special arrangement with Uni Key Health Systems and my office, you may purchase

111

the Doulton Ceramic Filter either by phone at 1-800-888-4353 or online at www.unikeyhealth.com.

- If you hike, camp, ski, or swim, never drink out of brooks, reservoirs, ponds, streams, or lakes, no matter how pristine or remote they may seem. Water must be boiled or filtered.
- If backpacking, camping out, or traveling in mountainous regions of the United States or abroad, invest in a portable water filter designed to filter our giardia cysts. A fine-pore filter of not more than three microns is desirable. Charcoal filters must contain a fine-pore filter. Portable drinking-water filters that remove giardia include General Ecology First Need, and the Timberline Filter; these filters can be purchased at outdoor and camping stores. The Katadyn is one of the best portable pocket filters on the market and has been used by the North Atlantic Treaty Organization (NATO). It can be purchased from Provisions Unlimited, P.O. Box 456, Oakland, Maine 04963. It weighs about 23 ounces and so is fairly lightweight as well as extremely efficient, with a pore filter of two microns. The other filters can be purchased at outdoor and camping stores.

food handling

Parasite infection can be avoided by treating all foods in a special cleansing bath. To remove parasites as well as sprays, fungi, and bacteria from food, soak all meat, fish, lamb, eggs, vegetables, and fruit thoroughly according to the following procedure:

1. Use half a teaspoon of Clorox to one gallon of water, obtained from your usual source. (To ensure that you are using the proper preparation, Dr. Hazel Parcells recommends that you use only the brand-name bleach Clorox.) Make sure to be careful when using bleach. At full strength, it is a powerful chemical.
2. Place the foods to be treated into the bath according to the following chart. Make a separate bath for each grouping.

Food Group	Treatment Time
Leafy vegetables	15 minutes
Root vegetables, thick-skinned vegetables, fibrous vegetables	30 minutes
Thin-skinned berries, peaches, apricots, plums	15 minutes
Thick-skinned fruits such as apples, citrus, bananas	30 minutes
Chicken, fish, meats, eggs (Each protein food should be treated in its own bath.)	20 minutes

Note: Meats can be thawed in a Clorox bath. The timing is about twenty minutes for a weight between two and five pounds. Frozen turkey or chicken should remain in the Clorox bath until thawed. Ground meats, of course, cannot be treated this way.

3. Remove foods from the Clorox bath and place into clear water for ten minutes. This is the rinse bath. Finish cleaning, dry all foods thoroughly, and store.

• If you choose not to use Clorox, freeze fish at −18°C for at least 48 hours to kill larvae. Freeze beef and pork at −20°C for at least 24 hours to kill larvae.

• To ensure 100 percent parasite-proof food, consider investing in cookware by Royal Prestige. Food is cooked by the minimum moisture method at 180°F—the temperature that kills germs, bacteria, and parasites, not vitamins and minerals. Royal Prestige is available through Uni Key, which may be contacted at 1-800-888-4353.

• When cooking meat in a conventional oven, always set the temperature to at least 325°F. The use of a meat thermometer is suggested when cooking in conventional ovens, and the internal temperature should be checked in several places. Beef should be cooked to an internal temperature of at least 160°F; lamb, veal, and pork to 170°F. Check for doneness always—i.e., no pink—especially in the center.

- When cooking meat or fish in a microwave oven, be aware that microwaves heat unevenly. Be sure to check the internal temperature in many different places. Fish must be heated to an internal temperature of 140°F for at least five minutes.
- In conventional ovens, cook fish until it's flaky and white. Bake at 400°F, eight to ten minutes per inch of thickness.
- It is best to buy your seafood from established dealers rather than from roadside stands or trucks.
- Use a mild bleach solution to clean all cooking utensils, cutting boards (particularly if they are wooden where bacteria can easily be trapped), or surfaces that have come in contact with uncooked foods.
- Avoid the habit of sampling dishes like sausage and gefilte fish before they are thoroughly cooked.
- Try to eat Pacific salmon and/or Pacific rockfish (red snapper) that has been commercially blast-frozen. If you eat sushi, avoid any that has been made from Pacific salmon and Pacific rockfish. These are known to contain parasites. Ask that your fish market carry blast-frozen fish.
- Unless you are an experienced sushi chef, it is best not to prepare raw fish dishes like sushi and sashimi at home. Experienced chefs are highly trained to know which fish species can be infected, and they can spot larvae.
- A food safety hotline sponsored by the Alliance for Food and Fibers Food Safety Information is available. Call 1-800-266-0200 with your questions.
- Maintain a balanced diet with moderate amounts of protein, high fiber, natural complex carbohydrates (such as beans, starchy root vegetables), and a variety of whole grains. Use lots of garlic in cooking. Snack on pumpkin seeds. Remember that parasites thrive on sweets and simple carbohydrates, so limit even natural sources of sugar from fruit and fruit juice, for example, to two or three portions a day. Natural oils in the form of unprocessed, expeller pressed safflower, sunflower, corn, flax, and sesame

can strengthen the immune system by fortifying the cell membrane walls. Please refer to my book *Eat Fat, Lose Weight* (Keats, 1999) for more information on the importance of essential fat in the diet for general overall health. (The book also contains menu ideas, shopping lists, food portion guides, and recipes for maintaining good health.)

- Use an unrefined natural sea salt in cooking. Salt has an antiseptic effect on body tissues.
- When eating out, skip the salad bars. Order only well-cooked food.
- Cook with lots of garlic, which contains natural antibiotic properties.
- Snack on pumpkin seeds, which have antiparasitic properties.
- Avoid sugar and other simple carbohydrates. Parasites thrive on them. Also, limit certain complex carbohydrates like potatoes, squash, whole wheat, and brown rice.
- Use unprocessed natural oils, such as expeller-pressed safflower, sunflower, corn, flax, and sesame, to help strengthen the immune system.
- Eat only well-cooked food.

travel arrangements

The enormous increase in worldwide travel may expose tourists to rare diseases. Pre-travel information on food, water, and other hygienic practices is recommended and can be obtained from The Traveler's Medical Service of Washington, D.C., at (202) 466-8109.

- When planning a trip abroad, be sensible and prepare well in advance. Contact the Traveler's Health Section of the Centers for Disease Control in Atlanta at (404) 639-3311 to obtain guides to regional diseases in the areas where you will be traveling.
- When traveling abroad or in mountainous regions of the United States where giardia thrives, take along your portable water filter or drink only from reliable bottled water sources. Eat only cooked or peeled fruits and vegetables.

- Avoid regional foods and special dishes that include raw, pickled, smoked, or dried fish, crabs, and crayfish. All beef and lamb should be thoroughly cooked.
- Consider taking along Pepto-Bismol as a diarrhea preventative. Take two ounces four times daily or one to two tablets four times a day for every day of travel. Dr. Ohhira's Probiotics 12 Plus (which doesn't need refrigeration) is a beneficial blend of friendly bacteria that can help prevent "traveler's diarrhea" or Montezuma's revenge.
- Bentonite, a clay-like liquid found in most health food stores, is a good natural parasite preventative. When taken in the morning and evening (at least one tablespoon each time), it has been known to protect travelers from disease by absorbing poisons in the intestinal tract and flushing them out of the system. My clients who are prone to diarrhea when they travel no longer are stricken after taking bentonite along.
- Avoid swimming in freshwater lakes.
- If you are sleeping in a tent in tropical areas, sleep under well-screened netting. Do not wear perfumes or after-shaves; they attract mosquitoes. Use insect repellent only.
- When traveling in the tropics, Africa, Asia, or the Middle East, stay covered up. Wear long sleeves and long pants. Be particularly careful at night. The anopheles mosquito that carries malaria comes out between dusk and dawn. You might also, in tropical climates, consider taking vitamin B_1 (about 50 to 100 milligrams per day) or brewer's yeast tablets (at least three tablets three times per day) to help naturally repel both fleas and mosquitoes from your body.
- Avoid using ice cubes made from tap water.
- Don't brush your teeth with tap water.
- Follow these same precautions with airline food.

sexual practices

Prevention of sexually transmitted parasitic disease depends on practicing safe sex and avoiding certain sexual practices.

- Regardless of sexual preference, wear condoms when engaging in sexual intercourse.
- Avoid oral-anal sex to prevent transmission of trichomonas, pinworms, ascaris, *Entamoeba histolytica,* giardia, and strongyloides.
- Avoid the use of sexual "toys" that may contain contaminated fecal matter.

animal care

Since household pets are nearly universally infected with certain parasites, every pet can be a source of infection.

- Be a "pooper scooper." Don't allow your dogs and cats to defecate on lawns and playgrounds, or in sandboxes. Collect and discard your animal's droppings. Feces should be burned or flushed whenever possible.
- Empty the kitty litter box daily. Gloves should be worn for this task. Feces should be burned or flushed down the toilet. Litter boxes should be cleansed frequently and disinfected with boiling water and a mild bleach solution. Pregnant women and immunocompromised patients in particular should wear disposable gloves and mask or, better still, relegate this responsibility to someone else.
- Keep animals outside the home if toddlers are in the house.
- Deworm all puppies and kittens on a regular basis. Some veterinarians suggest to begin at three and six weeks of age and continue with routine deworming every six months. Consult with your local veterinarian.
- Routinely check your animal's stool for worms yourself and then report to your vet.

- Have your veterinarian check for roundworm and tapeworm infections if the animal shows signs of illness or is rubbing its anus against the carpet or floor. Pumpkinseed-like particles found near the animal or where it has roamed are a sign of dog tapeworm.
- Consider keeping cats indoors to prevent their access to rodents and birds.
- Feed your pet cat or dog canned or dry food—or cooked (not raw) meat.
- Buy flea collars, or apply topical insecticides to dogs and cats to kill all fleas. A periodic flea bath may be necessary for thorough eradication.
- For a more natural approach, you might try adding fennel, rosemary, rue, or garlic to the animal's food to help repel fleas from the inside out. Garlic and yeast wafers are parasite- and flea-proof foods for your animals. Regularly disinfect your animal's food dish and water bowl with mild soapy water, then a diluted Clorox solution.
- To protect children playing in dirt from inadvertently ingesting soil contaminated with toxocara eggs, turn backyard soil under if your animal plays outside.
- Keep sandboxes covered.
- Provide your pet with filtered drinking water in a regularly cleaned container.
- Regularly brush and clean pets outdoors.
- Make sure all kitchen or dining room areas designed for food preparation or eating—i.e., countertops, tables, refrigerator, the dining room table—are strictly off-limits to your pets.

on the job

Many job-related activities can be a source of parasitic infection. Those whose jobs take them to developing countries for long periods of time are especially at risk.

- Overseas consultants, laborers, diplomats, and missionaries, as well as family members who accompany them, should be periodically examined with a complete blood count, liver function tests, and purged stool examination.
- All veterinary personnel, kennel workers, pet shop employees, animal trainers, sanitation workers, gardeners, zoo personnel, and cattle feedlot workers should be regularly checked for animal-transmitted infections.
- Check to see that your child's day-care center maintains good hygiene practices. All employees should routinely wash hands and scrub under the fingernails after using the bathroom and changing diapers. Children should be instructed in these good hygiene practices too. Toys and water faucets should be cleaned daily. Diaper changing should be relegated to one area, which should be cleaned after each changing with a soapy water solution. Children suffering from diarrhea should be kept at home.
- Every food handler in restaurants, hotels, and school or workplace cafeterias should be required to undergo stool testing. (We should all work to see that legislation for mandatory stool testing is enacted.)

at home

On the home front, there are often unsuspected risks for parasite infection that need closer scrutiny.

- Keep the home environment rodent-free to avoid exposure to rat tapeworm.
- In suburban and rural settings, watch out for raccoons. Their feces can be deposited in soil and objects that find their way into children's mouths. Raccoons carry roundworms, and over half may be infected. The Veterinary Medical Association has warned about the potential roundworm threat particularly, be-

cause small children chew and suck on objects that may be contaminated by raccoon feces in suburban neighborhoods.

- When employing a nanny, maid, or housekeeper, first screen her by using the questionnaire in Chapter Six. Use your judgment if you feel further medical testing is necessary. This is particularly important if this person is going to be preparing food for you and your family.

for women only

Women, because of their anatomical design, need to take special preventative measures.

- After urinating, wipe from front to back.
- When you have your yearly Pap smear, have the lab look for possible cervical pinworms and roundworms if you suspect a problem in the vaginal area or if you have frequent sexual relations with multiple partners.
- Be screened for toxoplasmosis if you are pregnant or attempting pregnancy.
- If pregnant, limit your exposure to cats. If possible, have someone else be caretaker of the household cat. Keep your pet away from your food and, in any event, have the cat checked for *Toxoplasma gondii*. Avoid undercooked meat.

Protecting you and your family from parasites involves a multifaceted approach. Old-fashioned common sense coupled with a heightened awareness and understanding of the methods of transmission and sources of potential infection are key factors in prevention. Our bodies are bombarded on a daily basis with a multitude of disease-producing bacteria, viruses, and allergens. The body's natural defender, our immune system, prevents us from "catching" germs and becoming host to every passing microbe.

I am reminded of the Ayurvedic (Indian) proverb that states, "If the field is barren, the seed, howsoever potent, may not be able to germinate."

In other words, parasites cannot infect a healthy body if the environment isn't conducive to them. Andreas Marx, a doctor of oriental medicine, said it best when he linked disease to "an imbalance of the body's terrain (pH, oxidation factor, and mineral balance)." We can stay healthy by nourishing our bodies with healthy food; supplementing our diets with immune-enhancing vitamins, minerals, and herbs; and by eliminating parasite risk factors from our environment.

10

closing comments

Without a doubt, parasitic infections are a reality in the United States today. One of the most outstanding parasitic hazards is contaminated water. Influxes of the highly infectious *Cryptosporidium parvum* and *Giardia lamblia* in water supplies throughout the country have sounded the alarm for proper filtration methods. Diaper-changing practices in our daycare centers has posed yet another threat of parasitic infections, with reports of nearly 20,000 cases of giardiasis annually. Add to all of this an increase in international travel, the rise of our country's immigrant population, the widespread use of antibiotics, high-sugar diets, and intrigue with exotic foods, as well as the practice of having multiple sexual partners. It's no wonder we're in parasitic jeopardy. Because there is sometimes no effective course of action for the treatment of these parasite-based disorders, prevention is most important. Trichinosis, for example, can be prevented by cooking meat to 170°F, but there is no therapy that has proven effective for treating this infection.[1] The animal-transmitted infection visceral larva migrans occurs most commonly in children who have pets or who play in areas that are frequented by dogs and cats. And since 60 percent of this country's 85 million households have a pet dog or cat, that puts literally millions of our children at risk. We can reduce this risk by following the guidelines in Chapter Nine, but there is no effective treatment for the respiratory and eye problems resulting from a visceral larva migrans infection.

But there is no need to become paranoid. We just need to become more responsible and conscious of a problem that many of us are not aware even exists. Parasites can only persist when they have a suitable environment. Diets high in sugars, refined carbohydrates, and fiber-depleted processed foods, and immune systems that have been weakened by these diets and by other environmental consequences of modern-day living, provide the ideal feeding ground for parasites. The problem is not so much "out there" as it is within our bodies.

On a national level, a great deal of energy and effort are directed toward educating the public regarding preventative measures for today's most threatening diseases—heart disease, cancer, AIDS. And more and more people are making lifestyle changes as public health education makes them aware of the risk factors related to these diseases—poor diet, environmental pollution, lack of exercise, smoking, drug and alcohol abuse, etc.

Heart disease, cancer, AIDS . . . these are not silent epidemics. The parasite problem, however, *is* a silent epidemic. There is a dangerous misconception that parasitic infections occur only in tropical areas or among the poor who live in unsanitary conditions. This misconception has resulted in a lack of awareness of the risk factors and symptoms associated with this insidious public health threat in America today. Furthermore, American doctors and other medical professionals have had so little training or experience with parasitic diseases that they are not alert to clinical symptoms. One of the most up-to-date clinical parasitology textbooks concludes:

The most important element in diagnosing a parasitic infection is often the physician's suspicion that a parasite may be involved—a possibility that is too often overlooked.[2]

The physician's lack of suspicion and concurrent underdiagnosis has left the public totally unaware of the scope of the parasite problem.

Making the matter even more complicated, the random stool examination—the standard method of detection used by most physicians who do routinely check for parasites—has proven to be insufficient and unreliable.

123

Unfortunately, based upon false negative results from inadequate testing procedures, most physicians rule out parasites as an underlying cause of disease. Since many symptoms of these infections are often non-specific and mimic other, more recognizable diseases, the condition is then misdiagnosed and health problems persist for months and sometimes even years before the real culprit is identified.

The study of parasitology in medical schools must be taken out of the departments of tropical diseases, because parasites are not just tropical anymore. All physicians, regardless of field of specialty, should be required to take basic courses in parasitology so that they suspect parasite-based disease when it is present and know how to effectively diagnosis it, treat it, and prevent its recurrence. We all must become responsible for the quality and safety of the food we eat and water we drink, for the way we handle our pets, for protecting ourselves when traveling, and for demanding appropriate medical testing and care when we suspect the possibility of parasitic infection.

Today, we are all susceptible to a wide array of parasite-related illness, ranging from rather common infections to rare disease manifestations. Our expanded travel opportunities and sanitation breakdowns on the homeland have exposed us to a surprising number of uninvited guests. *Guess What Came to Dinner?* provides some of the solutions to the chronic ill health Americans are experiencing as we enter the new millennium.

glossary

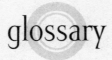

Acanthamoeba keratitis. A type of amoeba that causes corneal inflammation.

AIDS. Acquired immune deficiency syndrome. A disease of the body's infection-fighting system, thought to be caused by the HTLV–3 virus.

Alveoli. Air sacs in the lungs.

Amebiasis. An infection caused by internal animal parasites called amoebas.

Amoeba. Any of the protozoans of the genus *Amoeba* having an indefinite changeable form.

Anopheles mosquito. A mosquito belonging to the genus *Anopheles;* many transmit the malaria parasite to people.

Anorexia. Loss of appetite that leads to inability to eat.

Anus. The opening at the end of the alimentary canal through which solid waste passes.

Ascaris lumbricoides. Roundworm, the most common intestinal parasite.

Asphyxiation. Unconsciousness or death caused by lack of oxygen.

Asymptomatic. Exhibiting no symptoms.

Autoinfection. An infection that is caused by germs, viruses, or parasites that persist on or in the body.

Biopsy. Removal and examination, usually microscopic, of tissue from the living body. A biopsy is performed to establish a precise diagnosis.

Blastocystis hominis. Originally classified as a nonpathogenic yeast, blastocystis is now recognized as a protozoan.

Bloated. Swollen or puffed up, especially as with gas.

Bruxism. Continuous and unconscious grinding of teeth.

Caecum. The large pouch that forms the beginning of the large intestine.

Calabar. Refers to a temporary inflammatory reaction, known as Calabar swellings, characteristic of Loa loa infection.

Carcinoma. A malignant tumor originally comprising epithelial cells.

Cestoda. A class including the tapeworms.

Chorioretinitis. Inflammation of the retina and outer membrane of the eye.

Colic. Acute abdominal pain caused by spasm, obstruction, or distension of any of the hollow viscera.

Collagen. A protein comprising tiny fibers. It forms connective tissues such as tendons, ligaments, bone, and cartilage.

Complement Fixation Test (comp. fix. test). A test that measures those proteins in blood that are activated by infection.

Congenital. Present at birth but not hereditary.

Corneal ulcers. An inflammatory lesion of the structure that covers the lens of the eye.

Crohn's disease. An inflammatory bowel disease. The cause of this long-term illness is unknown.

Cryptosporidium. A protozoan known to cause diarrhea in both animals and humans.

Cutaneous. Of or pertaining to the skin.

Cutaneous larva migrans. Syndrome caused by dog and cat hookworm larvae and characterized by lesions on the skin at their point of entrance.

Cyst. A capsule that surrounds and protects the larval stage of some parasites.

Cysticerci. Cyst-like organisms.

Cysticercosis. A condition resulting from infection by pork tapeworm and characterized by seizures and brain deterioration.

Cystoscopy. Visual examination of the urinary tract with a special device called a cystoscope.

Dermatitis. Skin inflammation marked by redness, pain, and/or itching.

Disseminated strongyloides. A sometimes fatal condition caused by the nematode *Strongyloides stercoralis*.

Distension. Condition of being expanded due to or as if from internal pressure.

Duodenum. The shortest and widest part of the small intestine.

Dysentery. Infection in the lower intestinal tract that causes pain, fever, and severe diarrhea.

Ectoparasites. Parasites that live on the body (mites and tics).

Edema. Abnormal accumulation of fluid.

Elephantiasis. Enlargement and hardening of cutaneous and subcutaneous tissue, particularly of legs and scrotum; this condition is the result of lymphatic obstruction caused by a nematode.

Encephalitis. Inflammation of the brain.

Encyst. Become enclosed in a sac.

Endemic. Prevelant in or unique to a particular place or a particular people.

Endolimax nana. A type of very small amoeba that may be pathogenic and cause arthritis in people.

Endoparasites. Parasites that live inside the body.

Endothelial cells. Flat cells that line various cavities and vessels.

Entamoeba coli. A type of amoeba similar to *E. histolytica;* it may cause diarrhea but is not invasive of the colon mucosa.

Entamoeba hartmanni. An amoeba like *E. histolytica* but smaller.

Entamoeba histolytica. A variety of amoeba that is often responsible for causing an infection of the intestines or liver. (*See* amebiasis.)

Eosinophilia. An increase in the number of eosinophils in the blood.

Eosinophils. A type of white blood cell having two rounded projections, eosinophils comprise 1 to 3 percent of the total white blood cells. Allergies, some infections, and parasites can cause an increase in their numbers.

Epidemiologist. A person who studies epidemics and epidemic diseases.

Etiology. The study of causes or origins of disease.

Failure-to-thrive syndrome. Slowed growth in infants resulting from conditions that affect normal body functions, appetite, and activity.

Feces. Bodily waste excreted from the bowels.

Fibrosis. The overgrowth of fiberlike connective tissue.

Filariae. Microscopic roundworms.

Filariasis. Parasitic disease caused by *Filaria,* a type of worm.

Flocculation. A phenomenon relating to a suspension of finely divided particles in which the disperse phase separates in discrete, usually visible particles rather than in a continuous mass.

Flukes. Leaf-shaped flatworms.

Fluorescent Antibody Test (FAT). Test that reveals antibodies through the use of fluorescent lighting.

Giardiasis. Parasitic disease caused by *Giardia lamblia,* a protozoan.

Granulomas. Tumorlike masses.

Ground itch. Itchy patches of skin, pimples, and/or blisters resulting from infection by hookworm larvae.

Hemagglutination. The clumping of red blood cells into groups or masses.

Hematuria. A condition characterized by the presence of blood or red blood cells in the urine.

Hemoptysis. Spitting or coughing up of blood from the lungs or bronchial tubes.

Hepatic. Of or pertaining to the liver.

Hepatomegaly. Abnormal enlargement of the liver.

Histiocytes. Large cells in the reticuloendothelial system that have the ability to surround, eat, and digest small living things.

HIV. Human immunodeficiency virus. This virus attacks blood cells, resulting in suppression of the body's immune system and causing AIDS.

Hookworm. Small parasitic worms of the family Ancylostomatidae. With hooked mouths, these nematodes fasten themselves to the intestinal walls of their hosts.

Host. Organism that serves as the home for the parasite.

Hydrocephalus. A condition marked by an abnormal amount of spinal fluid in the head, enlargement of the skull, and compression of the brain.

Hyperglobulinemia. Excess of globulin in the blood.

Ileum. The portion of the small intestine that opens into the large intestine.

Immune response. Manner in which the body's defense system fights invasive bacteria, viruses, allergens, and parasites.

Immunoglobulin. Any of five antibodies found in the serum and external bodily secretions. Formed in response to certain foreign bodies (antigens).

Immunosuppressive drugs. Substances that reduce or halt immune response.

Infectious. Having the capacity to cause infection.

Intradermal. Within the layer of the skin that contains the nerve endings, sweat glands, and blood and lymph vessels.

Irritable bowel syndrome. Greatly increased movement of the intestines—both small and large—often associated with stress.

Lactose. Sugar found in milk.

Larva. The earliest stage of a newly hatched insect, often wormlike.

Leishmaniasis. An infection caused by a protozoan parasite that is transmitted by sand flies. It causes ulcers of nose, mouth, throat, and ears.

Lesion. A wound, injury, or circumscribed alteration of tissue caused by disease.

Leukocytosis. A significant increase in the number of white or colorless nucleated blood cells.

Leukopenia. Abnormal decrease in the number of white blood cells.

Lumen. The inner, open space in an organ.

Lymphangitis. An inflammation of one or more of the lymphatic vessels.

Lymphatic. Of or pertaining to the system of nodes and vessels that transport lymph, a bodily fluid that contains white blood cells and some red ones.

Malabsorption. Inadequate or defective absorbing of nutrients from the intestinal tract.

Megacolon. Abnormal and extensive widening of the large intestine.

Megaesophagus. Abnormal widening of the lower parts of the esophagus.

Methylene blue dye. Dye used in a lab test, helps contrast bacteria or parasites so that they are more easily seen.

Monocytes. The largest white blood cells; they are two to four times as large as red blood cells.

Moribund. Approaching death.

Mucosa. A membrane that lines bodily channels that communicate with the air.

Myocarditis. Inflammation of the muscle tissue of the heart.

Nematoda. The phylum name for unsegmented threadlike worms such as the hookworm.

Nephritis. Inflammation of the kidneys.

Night soil. Human excrement used as fertilizer.

Nodule aspirate. Removal of fluids from a nodule by suction.

Ocular larva migrans. Form of visceral larva migrans that infects the eye.

Onchocerciasis. Known as "river blindness," this condition is caused by the filaria *Onchocerca*.

Oocysts. The encysted form of some sporozoan eggs.

Papular. Characterized by small solid skin bumps.

Parasite. An animal or plant that grows, feeds, and is sheltered in or on another organism but contributes nothing to the survival of that host organism.

Parasitism. The condition in which an organism obtains its needs from another organism that it is living in or on it.

Parenchyma. The tissue that is characteristic of an organ rather than its supporting or connective tissue.

Pathogen. That which causes disease.

Perianal. About or around the anus.

Peritoneum. The membrane that covers the wall of the abdomen and is folded over inner organs.

Pernicious anemia. A disorder marked by inadequate production of red blood cells resulting from a nutritional deficit such as lack of iron, folic acid, or vitamin B_{12}.

Pinworms. *Enterobius vermicularis,* a nematode worm that infects the intestines and rectum.

Pleurisy. Inflammation of one or both of the membranous sacs that line the chest cavity and envelop the lungs.

Pneumocystic carinii. Parasite that causes a lung infection (pneumocystosis).

Pneumonitis. Inflammation of the lung.

Polymorphonuclear (PMN). White blood cell that is a granular leukocyte or neutrophil.

Porcine. Of or resembling pigs or swine.

Proglottids. A segment of a tapeworm that contains both the male and female reproductive organs.

Prophylaxis. Prevention or protective treatment.

Prostaglandin. A hormonelike substance found in various human body tissues. Prostaglandins may affect blood pressure, metabolism, and smooth muscle activity.

Protozoa. Single-celled organisms; the most primitive form of animal life.

Pulmonary. Of or pertaining to the lungs.

Roundworms. Of the phylum Nematoda, roundworms may be both parasitic or free living with muscles running the length of their bodies.

Schistosomes. Blood flukes.

Schistosomiasis. Infection caused by the *schistosoma* parasitic worm often found in water contaminated with human waste.

Scolex. Head of a tapeworm that attaches to the intestinal wall.

Scrotum. The external sac of skin that encloses the testes.

Serology. The study of antigen-antibody reactions in a test tube.

Sonogram. From *sono,* meaning sound. An image produced by ultrasonography, a sonogram is also called an echogram, sonograph, or ultrasonogram and is a technique in which sound waves are transmitted to hard-to-reach body areas and their echoes are recorded and studied.

Sputum. Material brought up from the lungs and coughed out.

Strabismus. Disorder of the eye muscles in which both eyes cannot be focused on the same point at the same time.

Striated muscle. Voluntary muscles comprising bundles of parallel fibers.

Strongyloides. A nematode or small roundworm.

Tapeworm. Long parasitic flatworm of the class Cestoda; inhabits the intestines.

Toxocaria canis. Dog roundworms that cause a disease called visceral larva migrans in humans, mainly children.

Toxocaria cati. Cat roundworms that cause a disease called visceral larva migrans in humans, mainly children.

Toxoplasma gondii. Intracellular parasite of birds and mammals (particularly cats) that can infect people.

Toxoplasmosis. Disease caused by _Toxoplasma gondii_, marked by tissue alteration in the brain and eye with lesions affecting the lungs, liver, heart, and muscles.

Trematoda. Leaf-shaped flatworms also known as flukes.

Trichomonas vaginalis. A parasitic protozoan that is widespread in humans. It lives in the vagina and sometimes causes inflammation, itching, and burning. It is also found in the male reproductive system.

Trophozoite. A protozoan of the Sporozoa class in the active stage.

Trophs. Short for trophozoite.

Ulceration. Development of a lesion on an internal mucous surface.

Vector. Agent that carries or transmits the infecting pathogen.

Vermifuge. A substance that expels or destroys intestinal worms.

Visceral larva migrans. A condition resulting from invasion of human viscera by nematode larva.

Volvulus. Intestinal obstruction caused by abnormal twisting.

Winterbottom's sign. A lymph condition at the base of the skull.

notes

Chapter 1:
"What You Don't Know *Can* Hurt You"

1. Centers for Disease Control, *Malaria Surveillance Annual Summary 1989*, issued November 1990.

2. L. Parrish, "The Protozoal Syndrome," *Townsend Letter for Doctors* (December 1990), 832.

3. "Technology, Funds Promise New Era in Parasitology," *Journal of the American Medical Association* 252 (December 14, 1984):3081.

4. Terry Kay Rockefeller, *Conquest of the Parasites,* produced by Paula Apsell, PBS, January 29, 1985, transcript, p. 8.

5. Centers for Disease Control, *Malaria Surveillance Annual Summary 1989*.

6. Jane Brody, "Test Unmasks a Parasitic Disease," *New York Times,* 26 October 1989, sec. B, p. 12.

7. L. Galland, et al., "Giardia lamblia Infection as a Cause of Chronic Fatigue," *Journal of Nutritional Medicine 1* (1990):27–31.

8. Parvel I. Yutsis, M.D., "Intestinal Parasites at Large," *Explore!* (1996):29.

9. Larry Parsons, "Child Contracts Parasite from Raccoon," *San Luis Obispo County Telegram-Tribune* (1998).

10. "Parasites in the United States Affect Millions," National Institute of Health (November 1, 1993).

11. Marilyn Chase, "Old Camper's Malady Now Strikes Often in City Settings," *Wall Street Journal* (April 28, 1997):B1.

12. P. W. Moser, "Danger in Diaperland," *In Health*, September–October 1991, 78.

13. *Ibid.*

14. William Blair, "Disease Is Cited in Veterans' Suit," *New York Times*, 24 July 1985, Sec. 2, p. 2.

15. Juan Walte, "Gulf War Parasite Halts Troop Blood Drive," *USA Today*, 13 November 1991, sec. A, p. 1.

16. M. Rosenbaum and M. Susser, *Solving the Puzzle of Chronic Fatigue Syndrome* (Tacoma, WA: Life Sciences Press, 1992), 51.

17. International Medical News Service, "Animal-Transmitted Diseases Often Unsuspected, Unrecognized," *Pediatric News* 11 (September 1977):9.

18. Larry Parsons, "Child Contracts Parasite from Raccoon," *San Luis Obispo County Telegram-Tribune* (1998).

19. C. Lane, et al., A Letter to the Editor, "If Your Uneaten Food Moves, Take It to a Doctor," *Journal of the American Medical Association* 260 (July 15, 1988):340.

20. J. McKerrow, et al., "Anisakiasis: Revenge of the Sushi Parasite," *New England Journal of Medicine* 319 (November 3, 1988):1228.

21. "Out, Damned Parasite!" ABCNEWS.com (May 22, 1997).

22. W. Petri and J. Ravdin, "Treatment of Homosexual Men Infected with *Entamoeba histolytica*," *New England Journal of Medicine* 315 (August 7, 1986):393.

Chapter 3:
"Guide to Parasites"

1. Alison Cook, "Unwelcome Guest, Reluctant Host," *Texas Monthly*, May 1985, 166–168.

2. Marilyn Chase, "Old Camper's Malady Now Strikes Often in City Settings," *Wall Street Journal* (April 28, 1997):B1.

3. D. P. Clark and C. L. Sears, "The Pathogenesis of Cryptosporidiosis," *Parasitology Today* (vol. 12, no. 6, 1996):221.

4. Omar M. Amin, "Seasonal Prevalence and Host Relationships of *Cyclospora cayetanensis* in North America during 1996," *Institute of Parasitic Diseases* (1996):2, 9.
5. "Out, Damned Parasite!" ABCNEWS.com (May 22, 1997).

Chapter 4:
"The Water and Food Connection"

1. Voge and John Markell, *Medical Parasitology,* 6th Ed., (Philadelphia: W. B. Saunders Co., 1986), 58.
2. "Special Report: Drinking Water's Hidden Dangers: Federal Regulations Revamped, but Serious Problems Still Exist," *USA Today* (October 21, 1998).
3. Moser, "Danger in Diaperland," 77–80.
4. J. H. Thompson, "Times, Manners, and the STD List: An Essay," *Laboratory Management,* July 1984, 16.
5. Jeanette K. Stehr-Green and Theodore Bailey, et al., "Acanthamoeba Kerititis in Soft Contact Lens Wearers," *Journal of the American Medical Association* 258 (July 3, 1987):57–60.
6. R. Gregory, et al., "Acute Schistosomiasis Among Americans Rafting in the Omo River, Ethiopia," *Journal of the American Medical Association* 251 (January 27, 1984):508–510.
7. Wilbur Cross and Thorleif Hellbom, "Long Journey to Nowhere," *Wide World,* February 1963, 85–134.
8. M. Wittner, "Eustrongylides—A Parasitic Infection Acquired by Eating Sushi," *New England Journal of Medicine* 320 (April 27, 1989):1124–1126.
9. Lane, "If Your Uneaten Food Moves, Take It to a Doctor," 340–341.
10. Shirley Mandel, "Nutrition for Better Health," *Jewish Press,* 8 April 1988, sec. M, p. 34–35.

Chapter 5:
"Man's Best Friend"

1. "Be My Hospital Buddy," *Medical Tribune,* March 25, 1987.
2. D. Elliot, et al., "Pet Associated Illness," *New England Journal of Medicine* 313 (October 17, 1985):985–995.

3. International Medical News Service, "Animal-Transmitted Diseases Often Unsuspected, Unrecognized," 9.
4. S. Bechtel, "What You Can and Cannot Catch from a Pet," *Prevention,* April 1984, 71.
5. Marjorie V. Baldwin, "We Love Animals, But . . ." *Wildwood Echoes,* Spring 1981, 3.
6. S. Teutsch, et al., "Epidemic Toxoplasmosis Associated with Infected Cats," *New England Journal of Medicine,* 300 (March 29, 1979):695–699.
7. R. McCabe and J. S. Remington, "Toxoplasmosis: The Time Has Come," *New England Journal of Medicine* 318 (February 4, 1988):313–315.

Chapter 7:
"Diagnosis"

1. S. Baron, editor, *Medical Microbiology, 3rd Edition* (New York: Churchill Livingstone, 1991), 1041.
2. *Ibid.*
3. Parrish, "The Protozoal Syndrome," 832–835.
4. Baron, 989.
5. L. Dowell, "Stool Examinations—A Procedure to Increase Their Value," *Official Journal of A.M.T.* (January–February 1961).
6. Brody, "Test Unmasks a Parasitic Disease," p. 12.
7. M. S. Wolfe, "Diseases of Travelers," *CIBA Clinical Symposia* 36 (November 2, 1984):28.

Chapter 8:
"Treatment"

1. D. Mirelman, et al., "Inhibition of Growth of Entamoeba histoyltica by Allicin, the Active Principle of Garlic Extract," *Journal of Infectious Diseases* 156(1):243–244, 1987.
2. "How to Fight Off Parasites and Pathogens—Safely," *Stool Scene,* Great Smokies Diagnostic Laboratory (January–March 1987):3.
3. D. L. Taren, and D. W. T. Crompton, "Nutritional Interactions During Parasitism," *Clinical Nutrition* (November–December 1989): 227–238.

4. D. Mahalanabis, K. N. Jalan, T. K. Maitra, S. K. Agarwal, "Vitamin A Absorption in Ascariasis," *American Journal of Clinical Nutrition* 29 (1976):372–375.

5. D. Mahalanabis, T. W. Simpson, M. L. Chakroborty, et al., "Malabsorption of Water Miscible Vitamin A in Children with Giardiasis and Ascariasis," *American Journal of Clinical Nutrition* 321 (1979):313–318.

6. E. P. Veriyam and J. G. Banwell, "Hookworm Disease: Nutritional Implications," *Reviews of Infectious Diseases* (1982):830–835.

7. Taren and Crompton, "Nutritional Interactions During Parasitism," 227–238.

8. *Ibid.*

9. C. Krakower, W. A. Hoffman, and J. H. Axtmayer, "The Fate of Schistosomes (*S. mansoni*) in Experimental Infections of Normal and Vitamin A Deficient White Rats," *Puerto Rico Journal of Public Health Tropical Medicine* 16 (1940):269–345.

10. R. E. Gingrich and C. C. Barett, "Effect of Dietary Vitamin A on the Innate Resistance of Cattle to Infestation by Larvae of *Hypoderma lineatum* (Deptera:Oestride)," *Journal of Medical Entomology* 12 (1975):13–15.

11. L. D. Stephenson, et al., "Relationships Between *Ascaris* Infection and Growth of Malnourished Pre-school Children in Kenya," *American Journal of Clinical Nutrition* 33 (1980):1165–1172.

12. G. Leitch, et al., "Dietary Fiber and Giardiasis," *American Journal of Tropical Medicine and Hygiene* 41(5):512–520, 1989.

13. "Giardiasis: An Update," *Infectious Disease Practice* 1 (1978):1–5.

14. Taren and Crompton, "Nutritional Interactions During Parasitism," 227–238.

15. *Ibid.*

16. "Keep the Bile Away From Giardia!" *Stool Scene,* Great Smokies Diagnostic Laboratory (Winter 1990):3.

17. "Drugs for Parasitic Infections," *The Medical Letter on Drugs and Therapeutics* (March 6, 1992):1.

18. Parrish, "The Protozoan Syndrome," 832–835.

Chapter 10:
"Closing Comments"

1. Baron, 966
2. *Ibid.*, 1126.

resources

Uni Key Health Systems
P. O. Box 7168
Bozeman, MT 59771
(800) 888-4353
From outside the U.S. (406) 586-9424
unikey@unikeyhealth.com
www.unikeyhealth.com

Distributor of Super GI Cleanse, Para-Key and Verma-Key products, undecylenic acid, Aqua Phase Homeopathic Yeast Formula, Dr. Ohhira's Probiotics 12 Plus, Parasite Test Kits, Water Filters, and Royal Prestige cookware.

Diagnostic Labs
Advanced Access Laboratory Inc.
Jeff Ingersoll—Client Relations Manager
21 Loop Road
Arden, NC 28704
(800) 328-7197

The GP-II panel includes parameters for digestion and absorption, as well as cultures for bacteria and yeast, and parasite testing. This is a fully certified medical diagnostic laboratory, specializing in the evaluation and diagnosis of gastrointestinal, nutritional, and metabolic disorders.

Consulting Clinical and Microbiological Laboratory, Inc.
333 Southwest 5th Avenue #620-7
Portland, OR 97204
(503) 222-5279

Provides stool microscopic exams as well as special stool culture for yeast.

Great Smokies Diagnostic Laboratory
18A Regent Park Boulevard
Asheville, NC 28806
(800) 522-4762

Specializes in multiple-sample testing, including traditional microscopy techniques for rectal mucus and purged and random stool, plus high-technology techniques such as immunoassay for specific parasite antigens. Great Smokies provides outstanding educational materials for both the general public and the medical profession.

Meridian Valley Clinical Laboratory
24030 132nd Avenue SE
Kent, WA 98042
(800) 234-6825

Features stool-sample testing with a special giardia antigen.

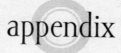

appendix

This section is a reprint of the March 2000 issue of *The Medical Letter*. It contains information your physician may find helpful in treating parasitic infections. There is a list of antiparasitic drugs as well as specific treatment dosages for particular infections.

The Medical Letter®

On Drugs and Therapeutics

Published by The Medical Letter, Inc. • 1000 Main Street, New Rochelle, N.Y. 10801 • A Nonprofit Publication

March 2000

DRUGS FOR PARASITIC INFECTIONS

Parasitic infections are found throughout the world. With increasing travel, immigration, use of immunosuppressive drugs and the spread of AIDS, physicians anywhere may see infections caused by previously unfamiliar parasites. The table below lists first-choice and alternative drugs for most parasitic infections. The manufacturers of the drugs are listed on page 157.

Infection	Drug	Adult dosage	Pediatric dosage
Acanthamoeba keratitis			
Drug of choice:	See footnote 1		
AMEBIASIS (Entamoeba histolytica)			
asymptomatic			
Drug of choice:	Iodoquinol	650 mg tid x 20d	30-40 mg/kg/d (max. 2g) in 3 doses x 20d
OR	Paromomycin	25-35 mg/kg/d in 3 doses x 7d	25-35 mg/kg/d in 3 doses x 7d
Alternative:	Diloxanide furoate*	500 mg tid x 10d	20 mg/kg/d in 3 doses x 10d
mild to moderate intestinal disease[2]			
Drug of choice:	Metronidazole	500-750 mg tid x 7-10d	35-50 mg/kg/d in 3 doses x 7-10d
OR	Tinidazole[3]*	2 grams/d divided tid x 3d	50 mg/kg (max. 2g) qd x 3d
severe intestinal and extraintestinal disease			
Drug of choice:[2]	Metronidazole	750 mg tid x 7-10d	35-50 mg/kg/d in 3 doses x 7-10d
OR	Tinidazole[3]*	600 mg bid to 800 mg tid x 5d	50-60 mg/kg/d (max. 2 g) x 5d
AMEBIC MENINGOENCEPHALITIS, PRIMARY			
Naegleria			
Drug of choice:	Amphotericin B[4,5]	1 mg/kg/d IV, uncertain duration	1 mg/kg/d IV, uncertain duration
Acanthamoeba			
Drug of choice:	See footnote 6		
Balamuthia mandrillaris			
Drug of choice:	See footnote 7		

* Availability problems. See table on page 157.
1. For treatment of keratitis caused by *Acanthamoeba*, concurrent topical use of 0.1% propamidine isethionate (*Brolene*) plus neomycin-polymyxin B-gramicidin ophthalmic solution has been successful (SL Hargrave et al, Ophthalmology, 106:952, 1999). In addition, 0.02% topical polyhexamethylene biguanide (PHMB) and/or chlorhexadine has been used successfully in a large number of patients (CF Radford et al, Br J Ophthalmol, 82:1387, 1998). PHMB is available as *Baquacil* (ICI America), a swimming pool disinfectant (E Yee and TK Winarko, Am J Hosp Pharm, 50:2523, 1993).
2. Treatment should be followed by a course of iodoquinol or paromomycin in the dosage used to treat asymptomatic amebiasis.
3. A nitro-imidazole similar to metronidazole, but not marketed in the USA, tinidazole appears to be at least as effective as metronidazole and better tolerated. Ornidazole, a similar drug, is also used outside the USA. Higher dosage is for hepatic abscess.
4. A *Naegleria* infection was treated successfully with intravenous and intrathecal use of both amphotericin B and miconazole, plus rifampin (J Seidel et al, N Engl J Med, 306:346, 1982). Other reports of successful therapy are questionable.
5. An approved drug, but considered investigational for this condition by the U.S. Food and Drug Administration
6. Strains of *Acanthamoeba* isolated from fatal granulomatous amebic encephalitis are usually susceptible *in vitro* to pentamidine, ketoconazole (*Nizoral*), flucytosine (*Ancobon*) and (less so) to amphotericin B. One patient with disseminated cutaneous infection was treated successfully with intravenous pentamidine isethionate, topical chlorhexidine and 2% ketoconazole cream, followed by oral itraconazole (CA Slater et al, N Engl J Med, 331:85, 1994).
7. A recently described free-living leptomyxid ameba that causes subacute to chronic granulomatous disease of the CNS. *In vitro* pentamidine isethionate 10 µg/ml is amebastatic (CF Denney et al, Clin Infect Dis, 25:1354, 1997). One patient, according to Medical Letter consultants, was successfully treated with clarithromycin (*Biaxin*) 500 mg t.i.d., fluconazole (*Diflucan*) 400 mg once daily, sulfadiazine 1.5 g q6h and flucytosine (*Ancobon*) 1.5 g q6h.

Infection	Drug	Adult dosage	Pediatric dosage
ANCYLOSTOMA caninum (Eosinophilic enterocolitis)			
Drug of choice:	Albendazole[5]	400 mg once	400 mg once
OR	Mebendazole	100 mg bid x 3d	100 mg bid x 3d
OR	Pyrantel pamoate[5]	11 mg/kg (max. 1g) x 3d	11 mg/kg (max. 1g) x 3d
***Ancylostoma duodenale*, see HOOKWORM**			
ANGIOSTRONGYLIASIS			
Angiostrongylus cantonensis			
Drug of choice:[8]	Mebendazole[5]	100 mg bid x 5d	100 mg bid x 5d
Angiostrongylus costaricensis			
Drug of choice:	Mebendazole[5]	200-400 mg tid x 10d	200-400 mg tid x 10d
Alternative:	Thiabendazole[5]	75 mg/kg/d in 3 doses x 3d (max. 3 grams/d)[9]	75 mg/kg/d in 3 doses x 3d (max. 3 grams/d)[9]
ANISAKIASIS (*Anisakis*)			
Treatment of choice:	Surgical or endoscopic removal		
ASCARIASIS (*Ascaris lumbricoides*, roundworm)			
Drug of choice:	Albendazole[5]	400 mg once	400 mg once
OR	Mebendazole	100 mg bid x 3d or 500 mg once	100 mg bid x 3d or 500 mg once
OR	Pyrantel pamoate[5]	11 mg/kg once (max. 1 gram)	11 mg/kg once (max. 1 gram)
BABESIOSIS (*Babesia microti*)			
Drugs of choice:[10]	Clindamycin[5]	1.2 grams bid IV or 600 mg tid PO x 7d	20-40 mg/kg/d PO in 3 doses x 7d
	plus quinine	650 mg tid PO x 7d	25 mg/kg/d PO in 3 doses x 7d
OR	Atovaquone[5]	750 mg bid PO x 7-10d	20 mg/kg bid PO x 7-10d
	plus azithromycin[5]	1000 mg daily PO x 3d, then 500 mg daily x 7d	12 mg/kg daily PO x 7-10d
***Balamuthia mandrillaris*, see AMEBIC MENINGOENCEPHALITIS, PRIMARY**			
BALANTIDIASIS (*Balantidium coli*)			
Drug of choice:	Tetracycline[5,11]	500 mg qid x 10d	40 mg/kg/d (max. 2 g) in 4 doses x 10d
Alternatives:	Iodoquinol[5]	650 mg tid x 20d	40 mg/kg/d in 3 doses x 20d
	Metronidazole[5]	750 mg tid x 5d	35-50 mg/kg/d in 3 doses x 5d
BAYLISASCARIASIS (*Baylisascaris procyonis*)			
Drug of choice:	See footnote 12		
***BLASTOCYSTIS* hominis infection**			
Drug of choice:	See footnote 13		
CAPILLARIASIS (*Capillaria philippinensis*)			
Drug of choice:	Mebendazole[5]	200 mg bid x 20d	200 mg bid x 20d
Alternatives:	Albendazole[5]	400 mg daily x 10d	400 mg daily x 10d
***Chagas' disease*, see TRYPANOSOMIASIS**			
***Clonorchis sinensis*, see FLUKE infection**			
CRYPTOSPORIDIOSIS (*Cryptosporidium*)			
Drug of choice:[14]	Paromomycin[5]	25-35 mg/kg/d in 2 or 4 doses	25-35 mg/kg/d in 2 or 4 doses

* Availability problems. See table on page 157.

8. Antiparasitic drugs can provoke neurologic symptoms, and most patients recover spontaneously without them. Analgesics, corticosteroids, and careful removal of CSF at frequent intervals can relieve symptoms (FD Pien and BC Pien, Int J Infect Dis, 3:161, 1999). Albendazole, levamisole (*Ergamisol*), or ivermectin have been used successfully in animals.

9. This dose is likely to be toxic and may have to be decreased.

10. Exchange transfusion has been used in severely ill patients with high (>10%) parasitemia (MR Boustani and JA Gelfard, Clin Infect Dis, 22:611, 1996). Combination therapy with atovaquone and azithromycin may be better tolerated (PJ Krause et al, American Society of Tropical Medicine and Hygiene Annual Meeting, 46:247, 1997, abstract 430). Concurrent use of pentamidine and trimethoprim-sulfamethoxazole has been reported to cure an infection with *B. divergens* (D Raoult et al, Ann Intern Med, 107:944, 1987).

11. Use of tetracyclines is contraindicated in pregnancy and in children less than 8 years old.

12. No drugs have been demonstrated to be effective. However, albendazole, mebendazole, thiabendazole, levamisole (*Ergamisol*) and ivermectin could be tried. Steroid therapy may be helpful, especially in eye and CNS infections. Ocular baylisascariasis has been treated successfully using laser photocoagulation therapy to destroy the intraretinal larvae.

13. Clinical significance of these organisms is controversial, but metronidazole 750 mg tid x 10d or iodoquinol 650 mg tid x 20d has been reported to be effective (DJ Stenzel and PFL Borenam, Clin Microbiol Rev, 9:563, 1996). Metronidazole resistance may be common (K Haresh et al, Trop Med Int Health, 4:274, 1999). Trimethoprim-sulfamethoxazole is an alternative regimen (UZ Ok et al, Am J Gastroenterol, 94:3245, 1999).

14. Treatment is not curative in immunocompromised patients and infection is self-limited in immunocompetent patients. Combination therapy with azithromycin 600 mg daily has been effective in some patients (NH Smith et al, J Infect Dis, 178:900, 1998). Nitazoxanide (an investigational drug in the USA manufactured by Romark Laboratories, Tampa, Florida, 813-282-8544, www.romarklaboratories.com) 500-1000 mg PO bid may be used as an alternative (J-F Rossignol et al, Trans R Soc Trop Med Hyg, 92:663, 1998). Duration of therapy is uncertain.

Infection	Drug	Adult dosage	Pediatric dosage
CUTANEOUS LARVA MIGRANS (creeping eruption, dog and cat hookworm)			
Drug of choice:	Albendazole[5]	400 mg daily x 3d	400 mg daily x 3d
OR	Ivermectin[5]	200 μg/kg daily x 1-2d	200 μg/kg daily x 1-2d
OR	Thiabendazole[15]	Topically	Topically
***CYCLOSPORA* infection**			
Drug of choice:	Trimethoprim-sulfamethoxazole[5,16]	TMP 160 mg, SMX 800 mg bid x 7d	TMP 5 mg/kg, SMX 25 mg/kg bid x 7d
CYSTICERCOSIS, see TAPEWORM infection			
***DIENTAMOEBA* fragilis infection**			
Drug of choice:	Iodoquinol	650 mg tid x 20d	30-40 mg/kg/d (max. 2g) in 3 doses x 20d
OR	Paromomycin[5]	25-35 mg/kg/d in 3 doses x 7d	25-30 mg/kg/d in 3 doses x 7d
OR	Tetracycline[5,11]	500 mg qid x 10d	40 mg/kg/d (max. 2g) in 4 doses x 10d
Diphyllobothrium latum, see TAPEWORM infection			
***DRACUNCULUS* medinensis (guinea worm) infection**			
Drug of choice:	Metronidazole[5,17]	250 mg tid x 10d	25 mg/kg/d (max. 750 mg) in 3 doses x 10d
Echinococcus, see TAPEWORM infection			
Entamoeba histolytica, see AMEBIASIS			
***ENTAMOEBA* polecki infection**			
Drug of choice:	Metronidazole[5]	750 mg tid x 10d	35-50 mg/kg/d in 3 doses x 10d
***ENTEROBIUS* vermicularis (pinworm) infection**			
Drug of choice:	Pyrantel pamoate	11 mg/kg base once (max. 1 gram); repeat in 2 weeks	11 mg/kg once (max. 1 gram); repeat in 2 weeks
OR	Mebendazole	100 mg once; repeat in 2 weeks	100 mg once; repeat in 2 weeks
OR	Albendazole[5]	400 mg once; repeat in 2 weeks	400 mg once; repeat in 2 weeks
Fasciola hepatica, see FLUKE infection			
FILARIASIS			
Wuchereria bancrofti, Brugia malayi			
Drug of choice:[18,19]	Diethylcarbamazine[20]*	Day 1: 50 mg, p.c. Day 2: 50 mg tid Day 3: 100 mg tid Days 4 through 14: 6 mg/kg/d in 3 doses	Day 1: 1 mg/kg p.c. Day 2: 1 mg/kg tid Day 3: 1-2 mg/kg tid Days 4 through 14: 6 mg/kg/d in 3 doses
Loa loa			
Drug of choice:[19,21]	Diethylcarbamazine[20]*	Day 1: 50 mg p.c. Day 2: 50 mg tid Day 3: 100 mg tid Days 4 through 21: 9 mg/kg/d in 3 doses	Day 1: 1 mg/kg p.c. Day 2: 1 mg/kg tid Day 3: 1-2 mg/kg tid Days 4 through 21: 9 mg/kg/d in 3 doses
Mansonella ozzardi			
Drug of choice:	See footnote 22		
Mansonella perstans			
Drug of choice:	Mebendazole[5]	100 mg bid x 30d	100 mg bid x 30d
OR	Albendazole[5]	400 mg bid x 10d	400 mg bid x 10d

* Availability problems. See table on page 157.

15. HD Davis et al, Arch Dermatol, 129:588, 1993.

16. HIV infected patients may need higher dosage and long-term maintenance.

17. Not curative, but decreases inflammation and facilitates removing the worm. Mebendazole 400-800 mg/d for 6d has been reported to kill the worm directly.

18. A single dose of ivermectin, 200 μg/kg, is effective for treatment of microfilaremia but does not kill the adult worm. In a limited study, single-dose diethylcarbamazine (6 mg/kg) was as macrofilaricidal as a multi-dose regimen against *W. bancrofti* (J Norões et al, Trans R Soc Trop Med Hyg, 91:78, 1997).

19. Antihistamines or corticosteroids may be required to decrease allergic reactions due to disintegration of microfilariae in treatment of filarial infections, especially those caused by *Loa loa.*

20. For patients with no microfilariae in the blood, full doses can be given from day one.

21. In heavy infections with *Loa loa,* rapid killing of microfilariae can provoke an encephalopathy. Apheresis has been reported to be effective in lowering microfilarial counts in patients heavily infected with *Loa loa* (EA Ottesen, Infect Dis Clin North Am, 7:619, 1993). Albendazole or ivermectin have also been used to reduce microfilaremia but because of slower onset of action, albendazole is preferred (AD Klion et al, J Infect Dis, 168:202, 1993; M Kombila et al, Am J Trop Med Hyg, 58:458, 1998). Albendazole may be useful for treatment of loiasis when diethylcarbamazine is ineffective or cannot be used but repeated courses may be necessary (AD Klion et al, Clin Infect Dis, 29:680, 1999). Diethylcarbamazine, 300 mg once weekly, has been recommended for prevention of loiasis (TB Nutman et al, N Engl J Med, 319:752, 1988).

22. Diethylcarbamazine has no effect. Ivermectin, 200 μg/kg once, has been effective.

Infection	Drug	Adult dosage	Pediatric dosage
FILARIASIS (*continued*)			
Mansonella streptocerca			
Drug of choice:[23]	Diethylcarba-mazine*	6 mg/kg/d x 14d	6 mg/kg/d x 14d
	Ivermectin[5]	150 µg/kg once	150 µg/kg once
Tropical Pulmonary Eosinophilia (TPE)			
Drug of choice:	Diethylcarba-mazine*	6 mg/kg/d in 3 doses x 14d	6 mg/kg/d in 3 doses x 14d
Onchocerca volvulus (River blindness)			
Drug of choice:	Ivermectin[24]	150 µg/kg once, repeated every 6 to 12 months until asymptomatic	150 µg/kg once, repeated every 6 to 12 months until asymptomatic
FLUKE, hermaphroditic, infection			
Clonorchis sinensis (**Chinese liver fluke**)			
Drug of choice:	Praziquantel	75 mg/kg/d in 3 doses x 1d	75 mg/kg/d in 3 doses x 1d
OR	Albendazole[5]	10 mg/kg x 7d	10 mg/kg x 7d
Fasciola hepatica (**sheep liver fluke**)			
Drug of choice:[25]	Triclabendazole*	10 mg/kg once	10 mg/kg once
Alternative:	Bithionol*	30-50 mg/kg on alternate days x 10-15 doses	30-50 mg/kg on alternate days x 10-15 doses
Fasciolopsis buski, Heterophyes heterophyes, Metagonimus yokogawai (**intestinal flukes**)			
Drug of choice:	Praziquantel[5]	75 mg/kg/d in 3 doses x 1d	75 mg/kg/d in 3 doses x 1d
Metorchis conjunctus (**North American liver fluke**)[26]			
Drug of choice:	Praziquantel[5]	75 mg/kg/d in 3 doses x 1d	75 mg/kg/d in 3 doses x 1d
Nanophyetus salmincola			
Drug of choice:	Praziquantel[5]	60 mg/kg/d in 3 doses x 1d	60 mg/kg/d in 3 doses x 1d
Opisthorchis viverrini (**Southeast Asian liver fluke**)			
Drug of choice:	Praziquantel	75 mg/kg/d in 3 doses x 1d	75 mg/kg/d in 3 doses x 1d
Paragonimus westermani (**lung fluke**)			
Drug of choice:	Praziquantel[5]	75 mg/kg/d in 3 doses x 2d	75 mg/kg/d in 3 doses x 2d
Alternative:[27]	Bithionol*	30-50 mg/kg on alternate days x 10-15 doses	30-50 mg/kg on alternate days x 10-15 doses
GIARDIASIS (*Giardia lamblia*)			
Drug of choice:	Metronidazole[5]	250 mg tid x 5d	15 mg/kg/d in 3 doses x 5d
Alternatives:[28]	Quinacrine[29]	100 mg PO tid x 5d (max. 300 mg/d)	2 mg/kg PO tid x 5d (max. 300 mg/d)
	Tinidazole*	2 grams once	50 mg/kg once (max. 2 g)
	Furazolidone	100 mg qid x 7-10d	6 mg/kg/d in 4 doses x 7-10d
	Paromomycin[5,30]	25-35 mg/kg/d in 3 doses x 7d	25-35 mg/kg/d in 3 doses x 7d
GNATHOSTOMIASIS (*Gnathostoma spinigerum*)			
Treatment of choice:[31]	Surgical removal		
OR	Albendazole[5]	400 mg bid x 21d	
GONGYLONEMIASIS (*Gongylonema sp.*)			
Treatment of choice:[32]	Surgical removal		
OR	Albendazole[5]	10 mg/kg/d x 3 d	10 mg/kg/d x 3 d
HOOKWORM infection (*Ancylostoma duodenale, Necator americanus*)			
Drug of choice:	Albendazole[5]	400 mg once	400 mg once
OR	Mebendazole	100 mg bid x 3d or 500 mg once	100 mg bid x 3d or 500 mg once
OR	Pyrantel pamoate[5]	11 mg/kg (max. 1g) x 3d	11 mg/kg (max. 1g) x 3d

* Availability problems. See table on page 157.

23. Diethylcarbamazine is potentially curative due to activity against both adult worms and microfilariae, but is not available in the US for this indication from the CDC. Ivermectin is only active against microfilariae.

24. Annual treatment with ivermectin 150 µg/kg can prevent blindness due to ocular onchocerciasis (D Mabey et al, Ophthalmology, 103:1001, 1996).

25. Unlike infections with other flukes, *Fasciola hepatica* infections may not respond to praziquantel. Triclabendazole (*Fasinex* – Novartis), a veterinary fasciolide, may be safe and effective but data are limited (R López-Vélez et al, Eur J Clin Microbiol, 18:525, 1999). It should be given with food for better absorption.

26. JD MacLean et al, Lancet, 347:154, 1996.

27. Triclabendazole may be effective in a dosage of 5 mg/kg once daily for 3 days or 10 mg/kg twice in one day (M Calvopiña et al, Trans R Soc Trop Med Hyg, 92:566, 1998).

28. Albendazole 400 mg daily x 5d may be effective (A Hall and Q Nahar, Trans R Soc Trop Med Hyg, 87:84, 1993). Bacitracin zinc or bacitracin 120,000 U bid for 10 days may also be effective (BJ Andrews et al, Am J Trop Med Hyg, 52:318, 1995).

29. Quinacrine is not available commercially, but as a service can be compounded by Medical Center Pharmacy, New Haven, CT (203-785-6818) or Panorama Compounding Pharmacy 6744 Balboa Blvd, Van Nuys, CA 91406 (800-247-9767).

30. Not absorbed; may be useful for treatment of giardiasis in pregnancy.

31. Ivermectin has been reported to be effective in animals but there are few data in humans (MT Anantaphruti et al, Trop Med Parasitol, 43:65, 1992; R Ruiz-Maldonado and MA Mosqueda-Cabrera, Int J Dermatol, 38:52, 1999).

32. M Eberhard et al, Am J Trop Med Hyg, 61:51, 1999

Infection	Drug	Adult dosage	Pediatric dosage

Hydatid cyst, see TAPEWORM infection

Hymenolepis nana, see TAPEWORM infection

ISOSPORIASIS *(Isospora belli)*

Drug of choice:	Trimethoprim-sulfamethoxazole[5,33]	160 mg TMP, 800 mg SMX qid x 10d, then bid x 3 wks	

LEISHMANIASIS (Cutaneous due to *L. mexicana, L. tropica, L. major, L. braziliensis;* mucocutaneous mostly due to *L. braziliensis;* visceral due to *L. donovani* [Kala-azar], *L. infantum, L. chagasi)*

Drug of choice:[34]	Sodium stibogluconate*	20 mg Sb/kg/d IV or IM x 20-28d[35]	20 mg Sb/kg/d IV or IM x 20-28d[35]
OR	Meglumine antimonate*	20 mg Sb/kg/d IV or IM x 20-28d[35]	20 mg Sb/kg/d IV or IM x 20-28d[35]
OR	Amphotericin B[5]	0.5 to 1 mg/kg IV daily or every 2d for up to 8 wks	0.5 to 1 mg/kg IV daily or every 2d for up to 8 wks
OR	Liposomal Amphotericin B[36]	3 mg/kg/d (days 1-5) and 3 mg/kg/d days 14, 21[37]	3 mg/kg/d (days 1-5) and 3 mg/kg/d days 14, 21[37]
Alternatives:	Pentamidine	2-4 mg/kg daily or every 2d IV or IM for up to 15 doses[38]	2-4 mg/kg daily or every 2d IV or IM for up to 15 doses[38]
OR	Paromomycin[39]*	Topically twice daily x 10-20d	

LICE infestation *(Pediculus humanus, P. capitis, Phthirus pubis)*[40]

Drug of choice:	1% Permethrin[41]	Topically	Topically
OR	0.5% Malathion[42]	Topically	Topically
Alternative:	Pyrethrins with piperonyl butoxide[41]	Topically	Topically
OR	Ivermectin[5,43]	200 µg/kg once	200 µg/kg once

Loa loa, see FILARIASIS

MALARIA, Treatment of *(Plasmodium falciparum, P. ovale, P. vivax,* and *P. malariae)*
Chloroquine-resistant *P. falciparum*[44]
ORAL

Drugs of choice:	Quinine sulfate	650 mg q8h x 3-7d[45]	25mg/kg/d in 3 doses x 3-7d[45]
	plus doxycycline[5,11]	100 mg bid x 7d	2 mg/kg/d x 7d
	or plus tetracycline[5,11]	250 mg qid x 7d	6.25 mg/kg qid x 7d
	or plus pyrimethamine-sulfadoxine[46]	3 tablets at once on last day of quinine	<1 yr: ¼ tablet 1-3 yrs: ½ tablet 4-8 yrs: 1 tablet 9-14 yrs: 2 tablets
	or plus clindamycin[5,47]	900 mg tid x 5d	20-40 mg/kg/d in 3 doses x 5d

* Availability problems. See table on page 157.
33. In sulfonamide-sensitive patients, pyrimethamine 50-75 mg daily in divided doses has been effective (JP Ackers, Semin Gastrointest Dis, 8:33, 1997).
34. For treatment of kala-azar, oral miltefosine 100-150 mg daily for 4 weeks was 97% effective after 6 months. Gastrointestinal adverse effects are common and the drug is contraindicated in pregnancy (TK Jha et al, N Engl J Med, 341:1795, 1999).
35. May be repeated or continued. A longer duration may be needed for some forms of visceral leishmaniasis.
36. Three preparations of lipid-encapsulated amphotericin B have been used for treatment of visceral leishmaniasis. Largely based on clinical trials in patients infected with *L. infantum,* the FDA approved liposomal amphotericin B *(AmBisome)* for treatment of visceral leishmaniasis (A Meyerhoff, Clin Infect Dis, 28:42, 1999; JD Berman, Clin Infect Dis, 28:49, 1999). Amphotericin B lipid complex *(Abelcet)* and amphotericin B cholesteryl sulfate *(Amphotec)* have also been used with good results. Some studies indicate that *L. donovani* resistant to pentavalent antimonial agents may respond to lipid-encapsulated amphotericin B (S Sundar et al, Ann Trop Med Parasitol, 92:755, 1998).
37. The dose for immunocompromised patients with HIV is 4 mg/kg/d (days 1-5) and 4 mg/kg/d on days 10,17,24,31,38. The relapse rate is high, suggesting that maintenance therapy may be indicated.
38. 4 mg/kg qod x 15 doses for *L. donovani;* 2 mg/kg qod x 7 or 3 mg/kg qod x 4 doses for cutaneous disease.
39. Two preparations of paromomycin have been studied. The first, a formulation of 15% paromomycin and 12% methylbenzethonium chloride in soft white paraffin for topical use, has been reported to be effective in some patients against cutaneous leishmaniasis due to *L. major* (O Ozgoztasi and I Baydar, Int J Dermatol, 36:61, 1997). The second, injectable paromomycin (aminosidine, not available in the USA), has been used successfully for the treatment of kala-azar in India where antimony resistance is common (TK Jha et al, BMJ, 316:1200, 1998).
40. For infestation of eyelashes with crab lice, use petrolatum. For pubic lice, treat with 5% permethrin or ivermectin as for scabies (see page 9).
41. A second application is recommended one week later to kill hatching progeny. Some lice are resistant to pyrethrins and permethrin (RJ Pollack, Arch Pediatr Adolesc Med, 153:969, 1999).
42. Medical Letter, 41:73, 1999.
43. Ivermectin is effective against adult lice but has no effect on nits (TA Bell, Pediatr Infect Dis J, 17:923, 1998).
44. Chloroquine-resistant *P. falciparum* occur in all malarious areas except Central America west of the Panama Canal Zone, Mexico, Haiti, the Dominican Republic, and most of the Middle East (chloroquine resistance has been reported in Yemen, Oman, Saudi Arabia and Iran).
45. In Southeast Asia, relative resistance to quinine has increased and the treatment should be continued for seven days.
46. *Fansidar* tablets contain 25 mg of pyrimethamine and 500 mg of sulfadoxine. Resistance to pyrimethamine-sulfadoxine has been reported from Southeast Asia, the Amazon basin, sub-Saharan Africa, Bangladesh and Oceania.
47. For use in pregnancy.

Infection	Drug	Adult dosage	Pediatric dosage

MALARIA, Treatment of *(continued)*
Chloroquine-resistant *P. falciparum (continued)*

Infection	Drug	Adult dosage	Pediatric dosage
Alternatives:[48]	Mefloquine[49,50]	750 mg followed by 500 mg 12 hrs later	15 mg/kg PO followed by 10 mg/kg PO 8-12 hours later (<45 kg)
	Halofantrine[51]*	500 mg q6h x 3 doses; repeat in 1 week[52]	8 mg/kg q6h x 3 doses (<40 kg); repeat in 1 week[52]
	Atovaquone[53]	500 mg bid x 3d	11-20 kg: 125 mg bid x 3d 21-30 kg: 250 mg bid x 3d 31-40 kg: 375 mg bid x 3d
	plus proguanil	200 mg bid x 3d	11-20 kg: 50 mg bid x 3d 21-30 kg: 100 mg bid x 3d 31-40 kg: 150 mg bid x 3d
	or plus doxycycline[5,11]	100 mg bid x 3d	2 mg/kg/d x 3d
	Artesunate* **plus** mefloquine[49,50]	4 mg/kg/d x 3d 750 mg followed by 500 mg 12 hrs later	15 mg/kg followed 8-12 hrs later by 10 mg/kg
Chloroquine-resistant *P. vivax*[54]			
Drug of choice:	Quinine sulfate **plus**	650 mg q8h x 3-7d[45]	25 mg/kg/d in 3 doses x 3-7d[45]
	doxycycline[5,11] **or plus**	100 mg bid x 7d	2 mg/kg/d x 7d
	pyrimethamine-sulfadoxine[46]	3 tablets at once on last day of quinine	<1 yr: ¼ tablet 1-3 yrs: ½ tablet 4-8 yrs: 1 tablet 9-14 yrs: 2 tablets
OR	Mefloquine	750 mg followed by 500 mg 12 hr later	15 mg/kg followed 8-12 hrs later by 10 mg/kg
Alternatives:	Halofantrine[51,55]*	500 mg q6h x 3 doses	8 mg/kg q6h x 3 doses
	Chloroquine	25 mg base/kg in 3 doses over 48 hrs	
	plus primaquine[56]	2.5 mg base/kg in 3 doses over 48 hrs	

---

* Availability problems. See table on page 157.

48. For treatment of multiple-drug-resistant *P. falciparum* in Southeast Asia, especially Thailand, where resistance to mefloquine and halofantrine is frequent, a 7-day course of quinine and tetracycline is recommended (G Watt et al, Am J Trop Med Hyg, 47:108, 1992). Artesunate plus mefloquine (C Luxemburger et al, Trans R Soc Trop Med Hyg, 88:213, 1994), artemether plus mefloquine (J Karbwang et al, Trans R Soc Trop Med Hyg, 89:296, 1995) or mefloquine plus doxycycline are also used to treat multiple-drug-resistant *P. falciparum*.

49. At this dosage, adverse effects including nausea, vomiting, diarrhea, dizziness, disturbed sense of balance, toxic psychosis and seizures can occur. Mefloquine is teratogenic in animals and should not be used for treatment of malaria in pregnancy. It should not be given together with quinine, quinidine or halofantrine, and caution is required in using quinine, quinidine or halofantrine to treat patients with malaria who have taken mefloquine for prophylaxis. The pediatric dosage has not been approved by the FDA. Resistance to mefloquine has been reported in some areas, such as the Thailand-Myanmar and -Cambodia borders and in the Amazon basin, where 25 mg/kg should be used.

50. In the USA, a 250-mg tablet of mefloquine contains 228 mg mefloquine base. Outside the USA, each 275-mg tablet contains 250 mg base.

51. May be effective in multiple-drug-resistant *P. falciparum* malaria, but treatment failures and resistance have been reported, and the drug has caused lengthening of the PR and QTc intervals and fatal cardiac arrhythmias. It should not be used for patients with cardiac conduction defects or with other drugs that may affect the QT interval, such as quinine, quinidine and mefloquine. Cardiac monitoring is recommended. Variability in absorption is a problem; halofantrine should not be taken one hour before to two hours after meals because food increases its absorption. It should not be used in pregnancy.

52. A single 250-mg dose can be used for repeat treatment in mild to moderate infections (JE Touze et al, Lancet, 349:255, 1997).

53. Atovaquone plus proguanil is marketed as a combination tablet in many countries and will soon be available in the United States (250 mg atovaquone/100 mg proguanil as *Malarone* – Glaxo Wellcome and 62.5 mg atovaquone/25 mg proguanil as *Malarone Pediatric*). The combination should be used only for acute uncomplicated malaria caused by *P. falciparum*. The dose of *Malarone* for 3-day treatment of malaria is 4 tablets daily in adults; 3 adult tablets daily for children 31-40 kg; 2 adult tablets daily for children 21-30 kg; and 1 adult tablet daily for children 11-20 kg. To enhance absorption, it should be taken within 45 minutes after eating (S Looareesuwan et al, Am J Trop Med Hyg, 60:533, 1999). Although approved for once daily dosing, to decrease nausea and vomiting the dose can be divided in two.

54. *P. vivax* with decreased susceptibility to chloroquine is a significant problem in Papua-New Guinea and Indonesia. There are also a few reports of resistance from Myanmar, India, Thailand, the Solomon Islands, Vanuatu, Guyana, Brazil and Peru.

55. JK Baird el al, J Infect Dis, 171:1678, 1995

56. Primaquine phosphate can cause hemolytic anemia, especially in patients whose red cells are deficient in glucose-6-phosphate dehydrogenase. This deficiency is most common in African, Asian, and Mediterranean peoples. Patients should be screened for G-6-PD deficiency before treatment. Primaquine should not be used during pregnancy.

Infection	Drug	Adult dosage	Pediatric dosage

MALARIA, Treatment of *(continued)*
  All *Plasmodium* except Chloroquine-resistant *P. falciparum*[44] and Chloroquine-resistant *P. vivax*[54]
    ORAL

Infection	Drug	Adult dosage	Pediatric dosage
Drug of choice:	Chloroquine phosphate[57]	1 gram (600 mg base), then 500 mg (300 mg base) 6 hrs later, then 500 mg (300 mg base) at 24 and 48 hrs	10 mg base/kg (max. 600 mg base), then 5 mg base/kg 6 hrs later, then 5 mg base/kg at 24 and 48 hrs

  All *Plasmodium*
    PARENTERAL

Infection	Drug	Adult dosage	Pediatric dosage
Drug of choice:[58]	Quinidine gluconate[59,60]	10 mg/kg loading dose (max. 600 mg) in normal saline slowly over 1 to 2 hrs, followed by continuous infusion of 0.02 mg/kg/min until oral therapy can be started	Same as adult dose
OR	Quinine dihydrochloride[59,60]	20 mg/kg loading dose IV in 5% dextrose over 4 hrs, followed by 10 mg/kg over 2-4 hrs q8h (max. 1800 mg/d) until oral therapy can be started	Same as adult dose
Alternative:	Artemether[61]*	3.2 mg/kg IM, then 1.6 mg/kg daily x 5-7d	Same as adult dose

  Prevention of relapses: *P. vivax* and *P. ovale* only

Infection	Drug	Adult dosage	Pediatric dosage
Drug of choice:	Primaquine phosphate[56,62]	26.3 mg (15 mg base)/d x 14d or 79 mg (45 mg base)/wk x 8 wks	0.3 mg base/kg/d x 14d

MALARIA, Prevention of[63]
  Chloroquine-sensitive areas[44]

Infection	Drug	Adult dosage	Pediatric dosage
Drug of choice:	Chloroquine phosphate[64,65]	500 mg (300 mg base), once/week[66]	5 mg/kg base once/week, up to adult dose of 300 mg base[66]

  Chloroquine-resistant areas[44]

Infection	Drug	Adult dosage	Pediatric dosage
Drug of choice:	Mefloquine[50,65,67]	250 mg once/week[66]	<15 kg: 5 mg/kg[66] 15-19 kg: ¼ tablet[66] 20-30 kg: ½ tablet[66] 31-45 kg: ¾ tablet[66] >45 kg: 1 tablet[66]
OR	Doxycycline[5,65]	100 mg daily[68]	2 mg/kg/d, up to 100 mg/day[68]
OR	Atovaquone/Proguanil[53]	250 mg/100 mg (1 tablet) daily[69]	11-20 kg: 62.5 mg/25 mg[69] 21-30 kg: 125 mg/50 mg[69] 31-40 kg: 187.5 mg/75 mg[69]
Alternative:	Primaquine[5,56,70]	30 mg base daily	0.5 mg/kg base daily

* Availability problems. See table on page 157.

57. If chloroquine phosphate is not available, hydroxychloroquine sulfate is as effective; 400 mg of hydroxychloroquine sulfate is equivalent to 500 mg of chloroquine phosphate.

58. Exchange transfusion has been helpful for some patients with high-density (>10%) parasitemia, altered mental status, pulmonary edema or renal complications (KD Miller et al, N Engl J Med, 321:65, 1989).

59. Continuous EKG, blood pressure and glucose monitoring are recommended, especially in pregnant women and young children. For problems with availability, call the manufacturer (Eli Lilly, 800-821-0538) or the CDC Malaria Hotline (770-488-7788).

60. Quinidine may have greater antimalarial activity than quinine. The loading dose should be decreased or omitted in those patients who have received quinine or mefloquine. If more than 48 hours of parenteral treatment is required, the quinine or quinidine dose should be reduced by 1/3 to 1/2.

61. NJ White, N Engl J Med, 335:800, 1996. Not available in the United States.

62. Relapses have been reported with this regimen, and should be treated with a second 14-day course of 30 mg base/day.

63. No drug regimen guarantees protection against malaria. If fever develops within a year (particularly within the first two months) after travel to malarious areas, travelers should be advised to seek medical attention. Insect repellents, insecticide-impregnated bed nets and proper clothing are important adjuncts for malaria prophylaxis.

64. In pregnancy, chloroquine prophylaxis has been used extensively and safely.

65. For prevention of attack after departure from areas where *P. vivax* and *P. ovale* are endemic, which includes almost all areas where malaria is found (except Haiti), some experts prescribe in addition primaquine phosphate 15 mg base (26.3 mg)/d or, for children, 0.3 mg base/kg/d during the last two weeks of prophylaxis. Others prefer to avoid the toxicity of primaquine and rely on surveillance to detect cases when they occur, particularly when exposure was limited or doubtful. See also footnotes 56 and 62.

66. Beginning one to two weeks before travel and continuing weekly for the duration of stay and for four weeks after leaving.

Infection	Drug	Adult dosage	Pediatric dosage

MALARIA, Prevention of *(continued)*
  Chloroquine-resistant areas[44]

Alternatives:	Chloroquine phosphate[65]	Same as chloroquine-sensitive	Same as chloroquine-sensitive
	plus pyrimethamine-sulfadoxine[46] for presumptive treatment[71]	Carry a single dose (3 tablets) for self-treatment of febrile illness when medical care is not immediately available	<1 yr: ¼ tablet 1-3 yrs: ½ tablet 4-8 yrs: 1 tablet 9-14 yrs: 2 tablets
	or plus proguanil[72]	200 mg daily	<2 yrs: 50 mg daily 2-6 yrs: 100 mg 7-10 yrs: 150 mg >10 yrs: 200 mg

MICROSPORIDIOSIS

Ocular (*Encephalitozoon hellem, Encephalitozoon cuniculi, Vittaforma corneae* [*Nosema corneum*])

Drug of choice:	Albendazole[5] plus fumagillin[73]	400 mg bid	

Intestinal (*Enterocytozoon bieneusi, Encephalitozoon* [*Septata*] *intestinalis*

Drug of choice:[74]	Albendazole[5]	400 mg bid	

Disseminated (*E. hellem, E. cuniculi, E. intestinalis, Pleistophora sp., Trachipleistophora sp.* and *Brachiola vesicularum*)

Drug of choice:[75]	Albendazole[5]	400 mg bid	

Mites, see SCABIES

MONILIFORMIS *moniliformis* infection

Drug of choice:	Pyrantel pamoate[5]	11 mg/kg once, repeat twice, 2 wks apart	11 mg/kg once, repeat twice, 2 wks apart

Naegleria species, see AMEBIC MENINGOENCEPHALITIS, PRIMARY

Necator americanus, see HOOKWORM infection

OESOPHAGOSTOMUM *bifurcum*
  Drug of choice: See footnote 76

Onchocerca volvulus, see FILARIASIS

Opisthorchis viverrini, see FLUKE infection

Paragonimus westermani, see FLUKE infection

Pediculus capitis, humanus, Phthirus pubis, see LICE

Pinworm, see ENTEROBIUS

---

* Availability problems. See table on page 157.

67. The pediatric dosage has not been approved by the FDA, and the drug has not been approved for use during pregnancy. However, it has been reported to be safe for prophylactic use during the second or third trimester of pregnancy and possibly during early pregnancy as well (CDC Health Information for International Travel, 1999-2000, page 120; BL Smoak et al, J Infect Dis, 176:831, 1997). Mefloquine is not recommended for patients with cardiac conduction abnormalities. Patients with a history of seizures or psychiatric disorders should avoid mefloquine (Medical Letter, 32:13, 1990). Resistance to mefloquine has been reported in some areas, such as Thailand; in these areas, doxycycline should be used for prophylaxis. In children less than eight years old, proguanil plus sulfisoxazole has been used (KN Suh and JS Keystone, Infect Dis Clin Pract, 5:541, 1996).

68. Beginning 1-2 days before travel and continuing for the duration of stay and for 4 weeks after leaving. Use of tetracyclines is contraindicated in pregnancy and in children less than eight years old. Doxycycline can cause gastrointestinal disturbances, vaginal moniliasis and photosensitivity reactions.

69. GE Shanks et al, Clin Infect Dis, 27:494, 1998; B Lell et al, Lancet, 351:709, 1998. Beginning 1 to 2 days before travel and continuing for the duration of stay and for 1 week after leaving.

70. Several studies have shown that daily primaquine beginning one day before departure and continued until two days after leaving the malaria area provides effective prophylaxis against chloroquine-resistant *P. falciparum* (E Schwartz and G Regev-Yochay, Clin Infect Dis, 29:1502, 1999). Some studies have shown less efficacy against *P. vivax*.

71. In areas with strains resistant to pyrimethamine-sulfadoxine, atovaquone/proguanil or atovaquone plus doxycycline can also be used for presumptive treatment. See page 6 for dosage.

72. Proguanil (*Paludrine* – Wyeth Ayerst, Canada; Zeneca, United Kingdom), which is not available alone in the USA but is widely available in Canada and overseas, is recommended mainly for use in Africa south of the Sahara. Prophylaxis is recommended during exposure and for four weeks afterwards. Proguanil has been used in pregnancy without evidence of toxicity (PA Phillips-Howard and D Wood, Drug Saf, 14:131, 1996).

73. Ocular lesions due to *E. hellem* in HIV-infected patients have responded to fumagillin eyedrops prepared from *Fumidil-B*, a commercial product (Mid-Continent Agrimarketing, Inc., Olathe, Kansas, 1-800-547-1392) used to control a microsporidial disease of honey bees (MC Diesenhouse, Am J Ophthalmol, 115:293, 1993). For lesions due to *V. corneae*, topical therapy is generally not effective and keratoplasty may be required (RM Davis et al, Ophthalmology, 97:953, 1990).

74. Octreotide (*Sandostatin*) has provided symptomatic relief in some patients with large volume diarrhea. Oral fumagillin (see footnote 73) has been effective in treating *E. bieneusi* (J-M Molina et al, AIDS, 11:1603, 1997), but has been associated with thrombocytopenia. Highly active antiretroviral therapy may lead to microbiologic and clinical response in HIV-infected patients with microsporidial diarrhea (NA Foudraine et al, AIDS, 12:35, 1998; A Carr et al, Lancet, 351:256, 1998).

75. J-M Molina et al, J Infect Dis, 171:245, 1995. There is no established treatment for *Pleistophora*.

76. Albendazole or pyrantel pamoate may be effective (HP Krepel et al, Trans R Soc Trop Med Hyg, 87:87, 1993).

Infection		Drug	Adult dosage	Pediatric dosage
PNEUMOCYSTIS carinii pneumonia (PCP)[77]				
Drug of choice:		Trimethoprim-sulfamethox-azole	TMP 15 mg/kg/d, SMX 75 mg/kg/d, oral or IV in 3 or 4 doses x 14-21d	Same as adult dose
Alternatives:		Pentamidine	3-4 mg/kg IV daily x 14-21 days	Same as adult dose
	OR	Trimetrexate	45 mg/m^2 IV daily x 21 days	
		plus folinic acid	20 mg/m^2 PO or IV q6h x 24 days	
	OR	Trimethoprim[5]	5 mg/kg PO tid x 21 days	
		plus dapsone[5]	100 mg PO daily x 21 days	
	OR	Atovaquone	750 mg bid PO x 21d	
	OR	Primaquine[5,56]	30 mg base PO daily x 21 days	
		plus clindamycin[5]	600 mg IV q6h x 21 days, or 300-450 mg PO q6h x 21 days	
Primary and secondary prophylaxis				
Drug of Choice:		Trimethoprim-sulfamethox-azole	1 tab (single or double strength) PO daily or 1 DS tab 3x/week	TMP 150 mg/m^2, SMX 750 mg/m^2 in 2 doses PO on 3 consecutive days per week
Alternatives:[78]		Dapsone[5]	50 mg PO bid, or 100 mg PO daily	2 mg/kg (max. 100 mg) PO daily
	OR	Dapsone[5]	50 mg PO daily or 200 mg each week	
		plus pyrimeth-amine[79]	50 mg or 75 mg PO each week	
	OR	Pentamidine aerosol	300 mg inhaled monthly via *Respir-gard II* nebulizer	>5 yrs: same as adult dose
	OR	Atovaquone[5]	1500 mg daily PO	

Roundworm, see ASCARIASIS

SCABIES (*Sarcoptes scabiei*)				
Drug of choice:		5% Permethrin	Topically	Topically
Alternatives:		Ivermectin[5,80]	200 µg/kg PO once	200 µg/kg PO once
		10% Crotamiton	Topically	Topically

SCHISTOSOMIASIS (*Bilharziasis*)				
S. haematobium				
Drug of choice:		Praziquantel	40 mg/kg/d in 2 doses x 1d	40 mg/kg/d in 2 doses x 1d
S. japonicum				
Drug of choice:		Praziquantel	60 mg/kg/d in 3 doses x 1d	60 mg/kg/d in 3 doses x 1d
S. mansoni				
Drug of choice:		Praziquantel	40 mg/kg/d in 2 doses x 1d	40 mg/kg/d in 2 doses x 1d
Alternative:		Oxamniquine[81]	15 mg/kg once[82]	20 mg/kg/d in 2 doses x 1d[82]
S. mekongi				
Drug of choice:		Praziquantel	60 mg/kg/d in 3 doses x 1d	60 mg/kg/d in 3 doses x 1d

Sleeping sickness, see TRYPANOSOMIASIS

STRONGYLOIDIASIS (*Strongyloides stercoralis*)				
Drug of choice:[83]		Ivermectin	200 µg/kg/d x 1-2d	200 µg/kg/d x 1-2d
Alternative:		Thiabendazole	50 mg/kg/d in 2 doses (max. 3 grams/d) x 2d[9]	50 mg/kg/d in 2 doses (max. 3 grams/d) x 2d[9]

*   Availability problems. See table on page 157.
77. In severe disease with room air PO$_2$ ≤ 70 mmHg or Aa gradient ≥ 35 mmHg, prednisone should also be used (S Gagnon et al, N Engl J Med, 323:1444, 1990; E Caumes et al, Clin Infect Dis, 18:319, 1994).
78. Weekly therapy with sulfadoxine 500 mg/pyrimethamine 25 mg/leucovorin 25 mg was effective PCP prophylaxis in liver transplant patients (J Torre-Cisneros et al, Clin Infect Dis, 29:771, 1999).
79. Plus leucovorin 25 mg with each dose of pyrimethamine.
80. Effective for crusted scabies in immunocompromised patients (M Larralde et al, Pediatr Dermatol, 16:69, 1999; A Patel et al, Australas J Dermatol, 40:37, 1999).
81. Oxamniquine has been effective in some areas in which praziquantel is less effective (FF Stelma et al, J Infect Dis, 176:304, 1997). Oxamniquine is contraindicated in pregnancy.
82. In East Africa, the dose should be increased to 30 mg/kg, and in Egypt and South Africa, 30 mg/kg/d x 2d. Some experts recommend 40-60 mg/kg over 2-3 days in all of Africa (KC Shekhar, Drugs, 42:379, 1991).
83. In immunocompromised patients or disseminated disease, it may be necessary to prolong or repeat therapy or use other agents. A veterinary parenteral formulation of ivermectin was used in one patient (PL Chiodini et al, Lancet, 355:43, 2000).

Infection	Drug	Adult dosage	Pediatric dosage

TAPEWORM infection — Adult (intestinal stage)

Diphyllobothrium latum (fish), *Taenia saginata* (beef), *Taenia solium* (pork), *Dipylidium caninum* (dog)

	Drug	Adult dosage	Pediatric dosage
Drug of choice:	Praziquantel[5]	5-10 mg/kg once	5-10 mg/kg once
Alternative:	Niclosamide	2 gm once	50 mg/kg once

Hymenolepis nana (dwarf tapeworm)

Drug of choice:	Praziquantel[5]	25 mg/kg once	25 mg/kg once

— Larval (tissue stage)

Echinococcus granulosus (hydatid cyst)

Drug of choice:[84]	Albendazole	400 mg bid x 1-6 months	15 mg/kg/d (max. 800 mg) x 1-6 months

Echinococcus multilocularis

Treatment of choice:	See footnote 85		

Cysticercus cellulosae (cysticercosis)

Treatment of choice:	See footnote 86		
Alternative:	Albendazole	400 mg bid x 8-30d; can be repeated as necessary	15 mg/kg/d (max. 800 mg) in 2 doses x 8-30d; can be repeated as necessary
OR	Praziquantel[5]	50-100 mg/kg/d in 3 doses x 30d	50-100 mg/kg/d in 3 doses x 30d

Toxocariasis, see VISCERAL LARVA MIGRANS

TOXOPLASMOSIS (*Toxoplasma gondii*)[87]

Drugs of choice:[88]	Pyrimethamine[89] **plus**	25-100 mg/d x 3-4 wks	2 mg/kg/d x 3d, (max. 25 mg/d) x 4 wks[90]
	sulfadiazine	1-1.5 grams qid x 3-4 wks	100-200 mg/kg/d x 3-4 wks
Alternative:[91]	Spiramycin*	3-4 grams/d x 3-4 wks	50-100 mg/kg/d x 3-4 wks

TRICHINOSIS (*Trichinella spiralis*)

Drugs of choice:	Steroids for severe symptoms **plus**		
	mebendazole[5]	200-400 mg tid x 3d, then 400-500 mg tid x 10d	200-400 mg tid x 3d, then 400-500 mg tid x 10d
Alternative:	Albendazole[5]	400 mg PO bid x 8-14d	400 mg PO bid x 8-14d

TRICHOMONIASIS (*Trichomonas vaginalis*)

Drug of choice:[92]	Metronidazole	2 grams once; or 250 mg tid or 375 mg bid PO x 7d	15 mg/kg/d orally in 3 doses x 7d
OR	Tinidazole[3]*	2 grams once	50 mg/kg once (max. 2 g)

* Availability problems. See table on page 157.

84. Patients may benefit from or require surgical resection of cysts. Praziquantel is useful preoperatively or in case of spill during surgery. Percutaneous drainage with ultrasound guidance plus albendazole therapy has been effective for management of hepatic hydatid cyst disease (MS Khuroo et al, N Engl J Med, 337:881, 1997).

85. Surgical excision is the only reliable means of treatment. Some reports have suggested use of albendazole or mebendazole (W Hao et al, Trans R Soc Trop Med Hyg, 88:340, 1994; WHO Group, Bull WHO, 74:231, 1996).

86. Initial therapy of parenchymal disease with seizures should focus on symptomatic treatment with anticonvulsant drugs. Treatment of parenchymal disease with albendazole and praziquantel is controversial and randomized trials have not shown a benefit. Obstructive hydrocephalus is treated with surgical removal of the obstructing cyst or CSF diversion. Prednisone 40 mg PO may be given in conjunction with surgery. Arachnoiditis, vasculitis or cerebral edema is treated with prednisone 60 mg daily or dexamethasone 4-16 mg/d combined with albendazole or praziquantel (AC White, Jr, Annu Rev Med, 51:187, 2000). Any cysticercocidal drug may cause irreparable damage when used to treat ocular or spinal cysts, even when corticosteroids are used. An ophthalmic exam should always be done before treatment to rule out intraocular cysts.

87. In ocular toxoplasmosis with macular involvement, corticosteroids are recommended for an anti-inflammatory effect on the eyes.

88. To treat CNS toxoplasmosis in HIV-infected patients, some clinicians have used pyrimethamine 50 to 100 mg daily (after a loading dose of 200 mg) with a sulfonamide and, when sulfonamide sensitivity developed, have given clindamycin 1.8 to 2.4 g/d in divided doses instead of the sulfonamide (JS Remington et al, Lancet, 338:1142, 1991; BJ Luft et al, N Engl J Med, 329:995, 1993). Atovaquone plus pyrimethamine appears to be an effective alternative in sulfa-intolerant patients (JA Kovacs et al, Lancet, 340:637, 1992). Treatment is followed by chronic suppression with lower dosage regimens of the same drugs. For primary prophylaxis in HIV patients with <100 CD4 cells, either trimethoprim-sulfamethoxazole, pyrimethamine with dapsone or atovaquone with or without pyrimethamine can be used (USPHS/IDSA, MMWR, Morbid Mortal Weekly Report, 48, RR-10:41, 1999). See also footnote 89.

89. Plus leucovorin 10 to 25 mg with each dose of pyrimethamine.

90. Congenitally infected newborns should be treated with pyrimethamine every two or three days and a sulfonamide daily for about one year (JS Remington and G Desmonts in JS Remington and JO Klein, eds, *Infectious Disease of the Fetus and Newborn Infant*, 4th ed, Philadelphia:Saunders, 1995, page 140).

91. For prophylactic use during pregnancy. If it is determined that transmission has occurred *in utero*, therapy with pyrimethamine and sulfadiazine should be started.

92. Sexual partners should be treated simultaneously. Metronidazole-resistant strains have been reported and should be treated with metronidazole 2-4 g/d x 7-14d. Desensitization has been recommended for patients allergic to metronidazole (MD Pearlman et al, Am J Obstet Gynecol, 174:934, 1996).

Infection	Drug	Adult dosage	Pediatric dosage
TRICHOSTRONGYLUS infection			
Drug of choice:	Pyrantel pamoate[5]	11 mg/kg base once (max. 1 g)	11 mg/kg once (max. 1 gram)
Alternative:	Mebendazole[5]	100 mg bid x 3d	100 mg bid x 3d
OR	Albendazole[5]	400 mg once	400 mg once
TRICHURIASIS (_Trichuris trichiura_, whipworm)			
Drug of choice:	Mebendazole	100 mg bid x 3d or 500 mg once	100 mg bid x 3d or 500 mg once
Alternative:	Albendazole[5]	400 mg once[93]	400 mg once[93]
TRYPANOSOMIASIS			
T. cruzi (American trypanosomiasis, Chagas' disease)			
Drug of choice:	Benznidazole*	5-7 mg/kg/d in 2 divided doses x 30-90d	Up to 12 yrs: 10 mg/kg/d in 2 doses x 30-90d
OR	Nifurtimox[94]*	8-10 mg/kg/d in 3-4 doses x 90-120d	1-10 yrs: 15-20 mg/kg/d in 4 doses x 90d; 11-16 yrs: 12.5-15 mg/kg/d in 4 doses x 90d
T. brucei gambiense (West African trypanosomiasis, sleeping sickness) hemolymphatic stage			
Drug of choice:[95]	Pentamidine isethionate[5]	4 mg/kg/d IM x 10d	4 mg/kg/d IM x 10d
Alternative:	Suramin*	100-200 mg (test dose) IV, then 1 gram IV on days 1,3,7,14, and 21	20 mg/kg on days 1,3,7,14, and 21
OR	Eflornithine*	See footnote 96	
T. b. rhodesiense (East African trypanosomiasis, sleeping sickness) hemolymphatic stage			
Drug of choice:	Suramin*	100-200 mg (test dose) IV, then 1 gram IV on days 1,3,7,14, and 21	20 mg/kg on days 1,3,7,14, and 21
OR	Eflornithine*	See footnote 96	
late disease with CNS involvement _(T.b. gambiense or T.b. rhodesiense)_			
Drug of choice:	Melarsoprol[97]*	2-3.6 mg/kg/d IV x 3d; after 1 wk 3.6 mg/kg per day IV x 3d; repeat again after 10-21 days	18-25 mg/kg total over 1 month; initial dose of 0.36 mg/kg IV, increasing gradually to max. 3.6 mg/kg at intervals of 1-5d for total of 9-10 doses
OR	Eflornithine	See footnote 96	
VISCERAL LARVA MIGRANS[98] (Toxocariasis)			
Drug of choice:	Albendazole[5]	400 mg bid x 5d	400 mg bid x 5d
	Mebendazole[5]	100-200 mg bid x 5d	100-200 mg bid x 5d

Whipworm, see TRICHURIASIS

Wuchereria bancrofti, see FILARIASIS

* Availability problems. See table on page 157.

93. In heavy infection, it may be necessary to extend therapy to 3 days.

94. No longer manufactured, but available from CDC in selected cases. The addition of gamma interferon to nifurtimox for 20 days in a limited number of patients and in experimental animals appears to have shortened the acute phase of Chagas' disease (RE McCabe et al, J Infect Dis, 163:912, 1991).

95. Suramin is the drug of choice for treatment of _T.b. rhodesiense_. For treatment of _T.b. gambiense_, pentamidine and suramin have equal efficacy but pentamidine is better tolerated.

96. Eflornithine is highly effective in _T.b. gambiense_ and variably effective in _T. b. rhodesiense_ infections. It is available in limited supply only from the WHO, and is given 400 mg/kg/d IV in 4 divided doses for 14 days.

97. In frail patients, begin with as little as 18 mg and increase the dose progressively. Pretreatment with suramin has been advocated for debilitated patients. Corticosteroids have been used to prevent arsenical encephalopathy (J Pepin et al, Trans R Soc Trop Med Hyg, 89:92, 1995). Up to 20% of patients fail to respond to melarsoprol (MP Barrett, Lancet, 353:1113, 1999).

98. For severe symptoms or eye involvement, corticosteroids can be used in addition.

MANUFACTURERS OF SOME ANTIPARASITIC DRUGS

albendazole – *Albenza* (SmithKline Beecham)

§ aminosidine, see paromomycin

§ artemether – *Artenam* (Arenco, Belgium)

§ artesunate – (Guilin No. 1 Factory, People's Republic of China)

atovaquone – *Mepron* (Glaxo-Wellcome)

atovaquone/proguanil — *Malarone* (Glaxo-Wellcome)

bacitracin – many manufacturers

§ bacitracin-zinc – (Apothekernes Laboratorium A.S., Oslo, Norway)

§ benznidazole – *Rochagan* (Roche, Brazil)

† bithionol – *Bitin* (Tanabe, Japan)

chloroquine HCl and chloroquine phosphate – *Aralen* (Sanofi), others

crotamiton – *Eurax* (Westwood-Squibb)

dapsone – (Jacobus)

† diethylcarbamazine citrate USP – (University of Iowa School of Pharmacy)

§ diloxanide furoate – *Furamide* (Boots, United Kingdom)

§ eflornithine (Difluoromethylornithine, DFMO) – *Ornidyl* (Ilex-Oncology, Inc)

furazolidone – *Furoxone* (Roberts)

§ halofantrine – *Halfan* (SmithKline Beecham)

iodoquinol – *Yodoxin* (Glenwood), others

ivermectin – *Stromectol* (Merck)

malathion – *Ovide* (Medicis)

mebendazole – *Vermox* (McNeil)

mefloquine – *Lariam* (Roche)

§ meglumine antimonate – *Glucantime* (Aventis, France)

§ melarsoprol – *Arsobal* (Aventis)

metronidazole – *Flagyl* (Searle), others

§ miltefosine – (Asta Medica, Germany)

§ niclosamide – *Yomesan* (Bayer, Germany)

† nifurtimox – *Lampit* (Bayer, Germany)

§ nitazoxanide – *Cryptaz* (Romark)

§ ornidazole – *Tiberal* (Hoffman-LaRoche, Switzerland)

oxamniquine – *Vansil* (Pfizer)

paromomycin – *Humatin* (Parke-Davis); aminosidine (topical and parenteral formulations not available in USA)

pentamidine isethionate – *Pentam 300, NebuPent* (Fujisawa)

permethrin – *Nix* (Glaxo-Wellcome), *Elimite* (Allergan)

praziquantel – *Biltricide* (Bayer)

primaquine phosphate USP

§ proguanil – *Paludrine* (Wyeth Ayerst, Canada; Zeneca, United Kingdom)

§ propamidine isethionate – *Brolene* (Aventis, Canada)

pyrantel pamoate – *Antiminth* (Pfizer)

pyrethrins and piperonyl butoxide – *RID* (Pfizer), others

pyrimethamine USP – *Daraprim* (Glaxo-Wellcome)

quinine sulfate – many manufacturers

§ quinine dihydrochloride

† sodium stibogluconate – *Pentostam* (Glaxo-Wellcome, United Kingdom)

*spiramycin – *Rovamycine* (Aventis)

† suramin sodium – (Bayer, Germany)

thiabendazole – *Mintezol* (Merck)

§ tinidazole – *Fasigyn* (Pfizer)

§ triclabendazole – *Fasinex* (Novartis Agribusiness)

trimetrexate – *Neutrexin* (US Bioscience)

---

* Available in the USA only from the manufacturer

§ Not available in the USA

† Available under an Investigational New Drug (IND) protocol from the CDC Drug Service, Centers for Disease Control and Prevention, Atlanta, Georgia 30333; 404-639-3670 (evenings, weekends, or holidays: 404-639-2888).

THE MEDICAL LETTER® (ISSN 1523-2859) is published and printed in the USA bi-weekly by The Medical Letter, Inc., a non-profit corporation. Second-class postage paid at New Rochelle, NY, and at additional mailing offices. POSTMASTER: Send address changes to THE MEDICAL LETTER at 1000 Main Street, New Rochelle, NY 10801-7537. ·Subscription fees: 1 year, $49.00; 2 years, $82.00; 3 years, $114.00 ($24.50—U.S. Funds—per year for individual subscriptions to students, interns, residents, and fellows in the USA and Canada; special fees for bulk orders). Major credit cards accepted. Subscriptions are accepted with the understanding that no part of the material may be reproduced or transmitted by any process in whole or in part without prior permission in writing.

Phone: 1-800-211-2769   Fax: 1-914-632-1733   WEB SITE: http://www.medletter.com

The Medical Letter • March 2000

index

INDEX